Dynamic Therapy of the Older Patient

Dynamic Therapy of the Older Patient

WAYNE A. MYERS, M.D.

A

Jason Aronson, Inc.
New York and London

Copyright © 1984 by Jason Aronson, Inc.

10 9 8 7 6 5 4 3 2 1

All rights reserved. Printed in the United States of America. No part of this book may be used or reproduced in any manner whatsoever without written permission from *Jason Aronson, Inc.,* except in the case of brief quotations in reviews for inclusion in a magazine, newspaper or broadcast.

Library of Congress Cataloging in Publication Data

Myers, Wayne A.
  Dynamic therapy of the older patient.

  Bibliography: p. 245
  Includes index.
  1. Aged—Mental health. 2. Psychotherapy. 3. Aged—Mental health—Case studies. 4. Psychotherapy—Case studies. I. Title. [DNLM: 1. Psychoanalytic therapy—In old age. WT 150 M996d]
RC451.4.A5M93   1984   618.97′68917   83-25772
ISBN 0-87668-623-4

Manufactured in the United States of America

To Joanne,
Tracy,
and Blake

Contents

Preface ix

1. Psychotherapy and the Older Patient 1
2. Therapy of a Lifelong Potency Problem 15
3. Therapy of an Alcoholic Woman 41
4. Therapy of a Virginal Woman 69
5. Therapy of a Depressed Man 107
6. The Dissolution of a Fifty-Year-Old Symptom 145
7. A Failed Psychotherapy in a Narcissistic Man 157
8. Assessment of General Treatability in the Older Patient 169

9.	The Impact of Losses on the Sense of Self	181
10.	The Impact of Retirement	191
11.	Dealing with the Loss of Love Objects	205
12.	Coming to Terms with Death	215
13.	The Therapist's Feelings	223
14.	The Usefulness of Dynamic Therapy with the Older Patient	237

References	245
Index	251

Preface

Interest in the treatment of the older patient has grown markedly in recent years. One of the recommendations of the Committee on Psychoanalytic Practice of the American Psychoanalytic Association (1980) was that population groups underserved by psychoanalysis, such as adults over the age of 50, should be reached. The Committee further noted that if the utility and feasibility of an analytic treatment approach could be demonstrated for such groups, then analytic services should be expanded to serve them. Similar assertions have also been made by the American Psychiatric Association (1981), which holds panels and discussion groups dealing with this area at its annual meetings.

In November 1982, the NIMH sponsored its first conference on aging, and a number of analysts made formal presentations. Many different issues of this period of life were considered, but a common request of the conference participants was for psychoanalytic studies of older individuals. This topic was covered at the December 1982 meetings of the American Psychoanalytic Association, with both a discussion group and a panel on the analytic treatment of the older patient. Unfortunately, there is little clinical material dealing with psychoanalyses of older patients (over the age of 50) in the psychoanalytic literature.

Since my personal experience with individuals over 50 demonstrates both the feasibility and the usefulness of employing the psychoanalytic method with such patients, I decided to present some of my significant clinical findings in this book.

Many recent medical advances have enabled individuals to live longer. Whether or not financial problems lead to a change in the long trend toward early retirement, older people are rapidly comprising an ever greater proportion of our society. Approximately 15 percent of the U.S. population is over 65 and nearly 25 percent is over 50.

Psychiatrically, we have not kept pace with the needs of this population. The predominant mode of interaction between doctors and older individuals has been through the prescription blank, rather than through any psychodynamically oriented interchanges. One of the aims of this book, therefore, is to correct this longstanding therapeutic bias.

Two important reasons for the neglect of this particular patient population by psychoanalysts and by psychoanalytically oriented psychotherapists involves Freud's specific interdictions against the analytic treatment of such patients and the issue of the strong countertransference feelings engendered during such treatments. As will be discussed, Freud (1898, 1904, 1905a) specifically cautioned against analyzing patients over 50, since he believed that such treatments were not feasible; our own reluctance as analysts to go counter to Freud's dicta in this area may make it difficult for us to investigate this "forbidden" territory. Alternatively, our own unresolved "transference" feelings toward Freud (our spiritual father), as well as any unresolved feelings toward our parents and our own analysts, which may be displaced onto Freud, may make it difficult for us to work with older patients.

It is likely that Freud's unresolved conflicts toward his own parents may have been partly responsible for his conclusions about the impracticality of treating older patients. Another way of characterizing Freud's difficulties here would be to lump his problems under the rubric of countertransference phenomena. I do not believe that Freud was alone in this regard: many analysts encounter a good deal of countertransference interference in their work with older patients.

With time, and the accumulation of data to the contrary by other analysts, the veracity of Freud's comments on this specific subject has been challenged, although relatively little has been published in this area. Only one case history of any length and detail (see Sandler 1978) and a few shorter ones exist in the psychoanalytic literature.

In this book, I review the important psychoanalytic articles dealing with the treatment of older patients. This is followed by six lengthy case histories of patients, four treated by psychoanalysis proper and two treated by psychoanalytic psychotherapy. The four analytic patients began their treatments at the ages of 54, 55, 59, and 62. The two psychotherapy patients began their treatments at the ages of 60 and 71. Not all these case histories are unmitigated success stories. Failures, as well as successes and partial successes, have been included.

In the case descriptions, I present some of the actual interpretive content of certain important sessions and some of the patients' responses to these interventions. In addition, I include some of my thoughts and feelings regarding both the timing and the content of certain of these interventions to illustrate how my normal analytic working capacity was affected by the countertransference difficulties I experienced; this is described in a chapter on the therapist's feelings. These examples, although sometimes uncomfortably revealing of my own psyche, seem to be necessary if this book is to illustrate the points I wish to make clearly and coherently.

A chapter on the assessment of analyzability in the older patient follows the case histories. I review some of the general factors that went into my assessments of the six individuals described, as well as some of the special features affecting the issue of analyzability in the older individual.

Subsequent chapters deal with developmental issues of importance in the older patient. Such topics as losses of aspects of the self, retirement and the "empty nest" syndrome, losses of love objects, and coming to terms with death are discussed. Pertinent data from the six cases are used to illustrate these discussions. In addition, an unusual phenomenon in the dreams of older patients is mentioned in the chapter dealing with loss of love objects.

It is my hope that this book will inspire psychoanalysts and psychoanalytically oriented psychotherapists to devote more time to the study and treatment of older patients.

Because of the intensification of many countertransference issues seen in the analyses of older patients (particularly for analysts and therapists who are younger than their patients), a challenging opportunity to review one's own analysis exists in work with such people; followed through, this will allow us to become better psychotherapists and psychoanalysts for all our patients. With an ever increasing older population, we also stand to be of considerable service to our society.

I would like to thank Dr. Leonard Diamond for his help in compiling a list of references on the subject of countertransference.

1
PSYCHOTHERAPY AND THE OLDER PATIENT

In my review of the psychoanalytic literature on the treatment of older patients, I found evidence that contradicts Freud's initial pessimism on the therapeutic efficacy of the analytic method for the over-50 patient.

The basis of the psychoanalytic dictum that the analysis of patients over 50 is contraindicated is found in three of Freud's early articles. In one (1898), he notes that analysis is not applicable to all cases. He then enumerates the limitations of the method and relates these to the maturity and understanding of the patient. He suggests that analysis is doomed to failure in people of advanced years because of the amount of material to be dealt with and the time required to do this. He sees the length of the treatment as precluding its usefulness in such patients, since they would have reached such an age that an improvement in their mental health would be of no real value.

In a second article (1904), Freud restricts his comments to patients over 50, noting that conditions for psychoanalysis are unfavorable over this age. He once again states that the amount of material to be dealt with is not manageable, as well as his feeling that the time required for such treatments would be inordinately long. He reiterated this position in a later paper (1905a) and spoke of the inelasticity of the mental processes and the ineducability of the older patient.

Nothing further appeared in the psychoanalytic literature on this subject for nearly 15 years, until Abraham (1919) wrote on psychoanalytic treatment of patients of an "advanced age" (meaning people in their forties and fifties). After agreeing with the overall correctness of Freud's views on the inefficacy of analytic treatment for older patients, he commented on the surprising degree of success he had obtained with a number of such patients (including individuals suffering from melancholic depression, obsessional neuroses, and agoraphobia) with the psychoanalytic method. He observed that his treatment failed with individuals who were essentially unable to speak of, and to integrate into their conscious awareness, material dealing with their instinctual lives.

Abraham went on to suggest that the prognosis in older patients was likely to be more favorable if the individuals had had a long period of successful sexual and social functioning after puberty; people who had never achieved such a period of successful functioning he saw as poor prognostic risks. He notes that such a prognosis also applies to younger patients and suggests that the duration of the neurotic process is probably more important in assessing prognosis in analysis than the age of the patient.

Two other points made by Abraham can be mentioned here: his recognition that the age of the patient does not preclude the patient's recovering childhood memories with the same degree of thoroughness that one might expect in a younger person and his introduction of a verbal parameter into the analyses of certain of his older patients. He notes that such analyses may differ from those conducted with younger patients. He seems to feel that certain older neurotic patients (especially obsessional neurotics) may need a greater degree of verbal input from the analyst—to stimulate and guide them—as they may have wished their fathers to have done in their childhood.

Following Abraham's article, nothing of consequence appeared in the psychoanalytic literature on this subject for nearly two decades. Then Kaufman (1937) described his "analytic" work with two, over-fifty, depressed patients. Although neither treatment appeared to be psychoanalytic, as Kaufman noted that the rule of free association could not be followed in either case, there are a number of points of interest in the paper. First, both patients improved after therapies several months in length. They also were found to have maintained their improvements in long-term follow-up. Second, Kaufman's patients were able to form potent transference relationships with him, which he likened to the transference neuroses of younger analytic patients. Third, he noted that the profound changes he was able to effect in a short time belied the contention that older individuals required inordinately lengthy treatments to modify their personalities.

Alexander (1944), in a discussion on the indications for psychoanalytic treatment, mentions two older men he saw. One, a man of 60 suffering from a phobic avoidance of venturing forth on the street, was not judged to be amenable to treatment when he would not accept any "trial interpretations" in the initial consultation, when the analyst endeavored to explain his phobia to him as being emotional, not physical. The other patient, a 66-year-old man with chronic alcoholism and spastic colitis, was not averse to dealing with the initial probes sent out by Alexander and was judged to be analyzable. No details of the treatments are provided, but it is of interest that Alexander determined the analyzability of the two men on their personality characteristics, not their respective ages.

Several papers on the treatment of older patients by Grotjahn (1940, 1951, 1955) offer little clinical material to document the conclusions presented, but Grotjahn's conclusions are of considerable interest. The only case cited in any detail in the three papers is that of a 71-year-old man suffering from senile dementia. The treatment was not analytic, since the couch and free association were not used, and transference had to be fostered by the therapist. No dream material was forthcoming and few childhood recollections were elicited. From this material, Grotjahn drew a parallel between the analytic situation seen with older patients and with children, when the analyst serves as a real object, and not simply as a transference object, for the patient.

In the first of the three articles (1940), Grotjahn follows Freud in seeing fear of death as an extension of fear of castration. He also comments on the importance of narcissistic losses for older people. He further suggests that narcissistic individuals have more difficulty dealing with the concepts of aging and death than have neurotic patients.

In the second of his three articles (1951), Grotjahn comments on the treatment of older people. He is the first analyst to note that the weakening of ego defenses in older individuals may actually facilitate their psychotherapy. He states that the limitations that reality imposes on narcissistic grandiosity is more acceptable to older than to younger individuals. He also sees older patients as having less difficulty in integrating interpretations than younger people have. Some of these observations presage Kernberg's (1980) observations, to be detailed later.

In the last of these articles (1955), Grotjahn comments on transference and countertransference issues in the treatment of older patients. He notes how older individuals often have to work through feelings of a reversed oedipal situation with their younger children. Again, he presages the comments of many later authors on the subject of envy in older patients, when he notes that parents should not envy their children, but should rather perceive in them their own continuity and immortality.

In the sphere of countertransference, he recognizes that unresolved hostility to one's parents, based upon prolonged submission to them in childhood, may cause the analyst to avenge himself on the older patient. He further notes that idealizations of older patients by the analyst may cover an underlying hostility. He also recognizes the need for the analyst to be strong enough to withstand the patient's hostility toward, as well as envy of, his youth.

Meerloo (1953, 1955) offers a number of observations. He underlines problems in self-esteem regulation in the aging patient, as well as the patient's increased sense of loneliness and his fear of death. In addition, he comments on the importance of narcissistic issues in such individuals and stresses the need of such patients to prove their potency in relationships with younger people.

Like Grotjahn before him, Meerloo (1953) notes that defenses may be weaker in the older patient, who may consequently respond more readily than younger ones to interpretations. He observes, however, that older patients may also find resolution of the transference relationship with the analyst difficult because the analyst may have become a real object in their lives, as well as a transference figure. He also describes the prominent countertransference attitude of many analysts who deny the idea of sexual pleasure in the older patient.

In his second article, Meerloo (1955) comments on the intensity of the transference relationships with such patients, with a combination of parental and filial images being transferred onto the person of the analyst. He also cites the frequency with which childhood memories are recovered and the prominence, or even the universality, in older people of dreams in which the attempt to deny the imminence of death is seen.

Hanna Segal (1958) was the first to cite clinical material from the analysis of an aging patient, although few verbatim transcripts of interactions between the patient and the analyst are detailed in her paper. Even here, the patient (a man in his mid-70's) was only seen in analysis for 18 months because he had to return to his native land. Follow-up, a year and one-half later, however, revealed him to be in good health.

Segal describes the transference relationship as a strong one. At various times, she represented the ideal father and son, as well as an idealized feeding mother. As the patient acknowledged his rage toward the important objects in his life, and toward the analyst, he began to recognize his fear of death and was able to tolerate his ambivalence toward his love objects. The end of the treatment came to symbolize approaching death for this patient, which was recognized as such and was freely spoken about.

Segal's patient saw his own imminent death as a reason for sorrow and mourning, and much positive analytic work was accomplished in this area. In addition, the patient was able to mourn other love objects in his life, and ended the treatment feeling that his life had been worth living. He no longer perceived his children and grandchildren as mere projections of himself, but rather saw them as separate objects, which he loved, and he was able to enjoy the thought of their living on and prospering after his own death.

In essence, Segal describes her patient's coming to terms with his own life and with his significant objects and being able to mourn his lost objects and his own imminent death. Thus, he could mitigate his envy of his progeny.

Erikson (1959) describes the basic task of the mature individual as the resolution of the polarity between integrity, on the one hand, and despair and disgust, on the other. Integrity is conceptualized in terms of accepting one's own life cycles and one's significant objects as inevitable and essentially as permitting of no replacements. It implies a love of one's family, without any wish for them to have been significantly different. When this is not successfully accomplished, Erikson finds that one sees prominent fears of death and feelings of despair because there is not enough time left in life to try alternative routes to the desired goal of integrity.

Melanie Klein (1963), in one of her final works, concentrates on the attenuation of excessive feelings of envy as a requirement for a relatively normal adaptation to old age. She notes that the individual who has identified with the pleasures and gratifications of other family members in childhood, without excessive envy, can usually identify with the satisfactions of the young in old age. Once more, we come across the concept that one must accept one's past and not suffer from too great a degree of envy to navigate the aging period successfully.

In a paper on narcissistic and object libido in the aged, Levin (1965a) speaks of the need to take quantitative factors into account when evaluating certain issues in older patients, such as the loss of a loved one. He particularly mentions high rates of change (concentrated losses within a unit of time) as predisposing the individual to emotional disturbances because of the degree of libidinal redistribution required before a state of equilibrium can once more be established.

Levin recognizes the difficulty some older individuals have in investing new objects, particularly when the old ones have not been sufficiently mourned. He believes that elderly individuals tend to become progressively self-centered and emphasizes the importance of separation from familiar surroundings and familiar objects in both the dream life and the emotional disorders of the elderly. As did Grotjahn (1955), Levin notes the prevalence of the reversed oedipal situation, whereby the child becomes the parent and vice versa, and the intense jealousy some older individuals show for younger members of the family. He also comments on the need of the older patient to be special in the eyes of the analyst, as a means of dealing with depletions in narcissism in aging.

A number of observations on aging and on the treatment of older patients are found in the three volumes put out by the Boston Society for Gerontological Psychiatry (1963, 1965, 1967).

Zinberg and Kaufman (1963) call for further studies of sexuality in the aged and note how difficult it is for younger psychiatrists to deal with this. They also note the difficulties attendant upon retirement for the elderly because of the self-esteem generally derived from a career. They further observe that many older persons need only a brief treatment, again contradicting Freud's early comments on such therapy. They tend to view aging as a developmental stage in life and comment sadly on how little emphasis is placed on the wisdom of older individuals in our youth-oriented culture. Also in this volume (1963), Goldfarb focuses on the difficulties some therapists have in dealing with the clinging dependency needs of some older patients.

Berezin (1963), in another paper in this volume, speaks of some of the problems facing the older patient (loss of love objects and retirement from a lifelong occupation) and of a need for regression in the aged because the need to achieve genital primacy may have diminished in the older individual. He envisions a need for older patients to retreat to earlier libidinal positions.

Again in this volume (1963), Kaufman emphasizes countertransference problems in the treatment of older individuals, and Linden (1963) discusses the idea of psychological "recession" in the older patient, by which he means the weakening of certain defenses. This is similar to Kernberg's (1980) notions, to be discussed later.

In a second volume in this series (1965), Cath refers to the increasing dependency needs of older patients as related to their loss of such "basic anchorages" as friendships and family ties. He describes a state of "omniconvergence," or a coming together of the personality, with an aura of peace, as being characteristic of the personality of the older individual. He observes that concomitant with the many object losses—a point Berezin (1965) also emphasizes —one may see a shift to attachments to transitional objects (money, photographs, etc.). In addition, Cath emphasizes the concept of depletion of resources in the older individual and the attendant need for restitutive measures to rebuild self-esteem, such as the idealization of children seen after a loss of narcissistic investment in the self. He compares the identity crises of old age with those of adolescence and conceptualizes such crises in terms of the individual's search for a more structured life.

Busse (1965) stresses the negative psychological effects of changes in perceptual acuity in older patients. Attitudes toward death and the need to prepare oneself for death are underscored in a discussion of some of the prior papers by Berezin et al. (1965). Levin (1965b) also notes the use of younger people as rejuvenating objects by older patients. When carried to an extreme, this may take on aspects of vampirism.

Gitelson (1965) describes an eight-month, twice-weekly psychotherapy with a 66-year-old woman who had been analyzed previously. He refers to sexual desires in this woman and the patient's capacity for an erotic transference. He also notes that the therapy was not especially different than one that might have been conducted with a younger patient. The treatment was interrupted by the patient because of her discomfort with the intensity of the transference, although she came back for follow-up visits and did reasonably well.

McMahon and Rhudick (1967), in an article from the third volume put out by the Boston Society for Gerontological Psychiatry, talk of reminiscing in the aged, viewing it as an adaptational response, based on their tests on 25 subjects of advanced age. They suggest that the high degree of reminiscing they observed may represent a reinvestment of the libido in an idealized image of the self in the past, in order to deal with the narcissistic mortifications of becoming older. They view such recollections of the past as a preparation for death and as a means of dealing with repeated object loss.

These findings are in contrast to those reported by the psychologist Giambra (1977), who tested 1,100 subjects (ages 17 to 92) with the Imaginal Processes Inventory, a long questionnaire about various types of daydreams. The questionnaire includes a subscale of questions about daydreams about the past. Giambra found no special tendency in the elderly, as compared with any other age group, to daydream more about the distant past.

Bibring (1966), in a paper on aging, views the period as a developmental–maturational phase of life. She notes that a number of important issues arise, such as termination of reproduction (which she sees as affecting self-esteem in men and the sense of their own physical attractiveness in women), termination of employment, object loss, physical illness, and death. She describes a number of fantasies associated with the idea of death and stresses the idea of a decrease in drive intensity in the aging. Finally, Bibring notes the assets of the aged person, such as the capacity to deal with ideas with little emotional bias.

Jacques (1970), whose writings were influenced by M. Klein, describes how the recognition of death in mid-life brings about a depressive reaction (seen as a reactivation of the early depressive position) that must be worked through again. This is accomplished by successfully resigning oneself to one's own imperfections, and to those in others, and by setting in motion the process of mourning for one's own death. His position is similar to that of Segal's (1958), whose work I described earlier. Again, it is primarily about the need for the older individual to mute excessive envy.

In one non-analytic article of interest in understanding the older patient, Neugarten (1970) refers to socially prescribed timetables for the ordering of major life events, as well as the individual's sense of timing—in other words, is the individual late or early or on time with regard to major life events? In a survey of 100 highly placed men and women who were asked what they regarded as the most salient feature of middle adulthood, both sexes spoke of having come to perceive time in a different way. They began to conceptualize their lives in terms of time left to them, not time already lived. They also spoke of their awareness of the finiteness of time. These perspectives were clearly related to their recognition of the imminence of death.

Neugarten further refers to women rehearsing for widowhood in middle age and men sponsoring their children or younger colleagues. She thus underscores the changed time perspective seen in the older patient and recognizes the need of the older individual to work through an envy of the young.

In a number of other studies cited by Neugarten, she and her co-workers noted that expectable events (the climacteric in women, retirement in men, or death in either sex) do not cause as much stress as unexpected events or events occurring at an unexpected time. For example, she noted that the prospect of death itself may not pose a crisis, whereas the idea of dying in an unfamiliar setting may.

She does not deny that expectable life events may be difficult for some older individuals, although she sees these individuals as being in the minority. She does emphasize that events that upset the rhythm of the life cycle or that occur out of sequence, such as the death of a parent in one's childhood, rather than later in life, or a late marriage, or the early or late birth of a child, are likely to be stressful.

Turning to case histories, Hurn (1969) reported an analysis of several years of a 50-year-old man. Although the patient left treatment, he derived marked benefit. Wolff (1971) reported on the treatment of 54 older patients (mean age 64 years) and suggested that memory disturbances were a significant obstacle to treatment.

The most detailed case history in the analytic literature, of the analysis of an older patient, is reported by Sandler (1978). She describes, at length, the analysis of a man from the ages of 58 to 66. She initially sees the need for adaptation in the aging individual and mentions the useful effect psychoanalysis can have upon this process.

The patient presented for analysis with a panic attack, essentially related to his unconscious fears of loss of control over his sexual and aggressive drive derivative wishes. Sandler notes the patient's concern with aging and with death and a defensive retreat from an unconscious fear of his own aggression into a position of having to please and placate narcissistically invested (idealized) objects, such as the analyst. Her formulations of the case are essentially those of the self psychologists (e.g., Kohut, 1971), as when she notes that the patient's early symptom of impotence is related to his perception of the difference between his real and his idealized self. She goes on to note how this self-confrontation, along with an awareness of aging and concomitant threats of helplessness and death, led the patient to experience a panicky fear of disintegration and somatic symptoms, which brought him into treatment.

In her description of the case, it appears that Sandler devoted her therapeutic interventions to issues involving the patient's narcissistic mortification, not to interpretations of the manifestations of transference. Thus, she describes how the patient decided to leave his job as an architect in order to study to be an English teacher so that he might teach immigrants. Sandler then notes the probable acting-out in this decision as, related to his identification with her as the immigrant he wished to teach English to, and then speaks of her intuitive feeling that it would have been incorrect to interpret the transference ramifications of the material. She further notes how she avoided oedipal interpretations, as she felt that the patient would have experienced them as an attack. Hence, she concentrated on the placatory and narcissistic aspects of his relationship with her. When the patient left his wife and formed a liaison with another woman, Sandler felt that to interpret the transference elements in this new relationship might have inhibited it by seeming to be critical and prohibiting. Similarly, she chose to concentrate on interpretations involving feelings of humiliation, rather than feelings of castration anxiety.

Finally, Sandler notes that the patient's mourning for his father helped him to prepare for his own old age and to mourn for his own past self. She sees his analysis as involving neurotic problems encapsulated within a narcissistic matrix and then observes that the oedipal elements in the case seemed muted, and were not as strong as they might have been had they appeared in a younger patient.

Shainess (1979) notes her surprise at the capacity for change in many of the middle-aged patients she treated. These individuals had had previous unsuccessful treatments and were suffering from serious psychosomatic problems, but they did well in treatment with her.

In three clinical vignettes from her analyses of older individuals, King (1980) brings up a number of theoretical points. She suggests that the successful treatment of middle-aged and elderly patients is determined by their re-experiencing and working through, in the transference relationship with the analyst, their adolescent traumata. She thus views the issues posed in both phases of life (adolescence and middle age) as being similar—for example, the need to deal with sexual and biological changes and problems of dependence and independence. She sees the breakdown of old defenses as leading to identity crises in both time epochs, which predispose to concomitant changes in the self-image and possible narcissistic mortifications.

King further notes how the awareness of changes in life situations introduces a sense of urgency into the analysis of middle-aged patients, which may help establish the therapeutic alliance to a degree often not seen with younger adults. Such patients are usually aware of the fact that this is their last chance to change their lives and their important object-relationships.

She further underscores the importance of transference and countertransference issues in the treatment of older patients, noting how intense the transference relationships are and the concomitant poignancy of the affects aroused in the analyst toward these patients. She points out the need to have come to terms with one's feelings for one's own parents and with one's own aging process.

She observes that the reality features of aging impose a time limit on the treatment and that there may be financial problems for individuals with a fixed income. She further remarks on how some older patients may deny the realistic time limitations imposed on them by age and may leave to the analyst the responsibility of carrying the sense of urgency of their situations. She also comments on the difficulties one may encounter when attempting to terminate such analyses, especially when the patient has the fantasy that by avoiding any real therapeutic change they may avoid both aging and death.

Kernberg, in *Internal World and External Reality* (1980), discusses both normal and pathological narcissism in middle age and the treatment of older patients. In a section on normal narcissism, Kernberg notes the role inversion that occurs between middle-aged parents and their young and adolescent children, with a consequent gain in understanding about one's own past and a heightened identification with one's own parents. He underscores the need to overcome oedipal guilt in order to accept this role reversal without experiencing an excessive degree of anxiety at what might be viewed as a triumph over an oedipal foe.

Kernberg further observes that, in middle age, we should begin to perceive our own limitations and begin to accept them. We must also begin to recognize the fact that other people are likely to achieve more in life than we have. Acceptance of these life limitations involves both the overcoming of oedipal problems and the working through of pre-oedipal envy. He also suggests that one must come to terms with the realistic limits, the mutability potential, imposed by one's character, and must accept these parameters maturely, without the rationalizations and denials so characteristic of the narcissistic personality. He notes that the ability to accept object losses and self-failures, while recognizing that one can meaningfully carry on a useful life is a key task of middle age. A final comment of importance concerns the extended mourning periods many individuals undergo for their parents and he suggests that such lengthy mourning may be a means of integrating oedipal conflicts into the personality.

In his chapter on pathological narcissism in middle age, Kernberg speaks of the tendency of narcissistic patients to devalue objects as a defense against envy, but at the price of a pervasive sense of emptiness. He notes that such individuals spoil success because of their relentless greed and that they never find lasting satisfaction. He also comments on the ingratitude narcissistic patients feel for what has been received in the past and their wish to recover what is no longer available to them. In other words, such people envy their own pasts.

Kernberg also notes how such patients often seduce younger people to help restore their own lost grandiosity. Such liaisons generally languish, however, because of the inability of such people to relate to others. Hence, the narcissistic patient is doomed to live eternally in the present, always reenacting a cycle of temporary idealizations and subsequent devaluations.

Kernberg also comments on how such narcissistic individuals envy the growth of their adolescent children. In particular, they attempt to maintain their own youth (through sexual liaisons and hypomanic business undertakings) to deny the anxieties aroused by aging and to escape from a normal mourning of the aging process. The realistic need for the support of, and dependence on, others induces shame and a sense of failure and humiliation that leads such people to devalue others (including the analyst) as a defense.

Narcissistic individuals tend to become greatly depressed in middle age, and may be more apt to accept psychoanalytic intervention. Kernberg sees these people as having a better prognosis at this age than earlier in their lives, having learned from experience the inefficacy of their narcissistic defenses. The impact of reality may thus enhance their self-awareness and the motivation for treatment.

Kernberg sees as most amenable to treatment in middle age individuals suffering from depression, regret, guilt, and remorse for wasted time and opportunities. Individuals who suffer from empty rage and who blame their difficulties on others have a more guarded prognosis.

2
THERAPY OF A LIFELONG POTENCY PROBLEM: Mr. T

Mr. T, a Jewish businessman, was 59 years old at the time that he was referred to me for treatment; and there was approximately a two-decade difference in our ages. The patient had been seen by his prior therapist, who had relocated his practice, in twice-weekly psychotherapy for a period of two years because of a lifelong potency problem. He had experienced difficulty in achieving and in maintaining an erection when he was in bed with a woman. On the very few occasions when intromission had been successful, he had ejaculated prematurely. Generally, however, ejaculation had occurred prior to entering the vagina.

His experience with his prior therapist was his third attempt at psychotherapy since his late 20's. Mr. T's first treatment experience, at 29, consisted of a few supportive sessions with a psychiatrist and some concomitant injections of testosterone from an internist. This attempt foundered after a few months and the patient did not enter therapy again until his sexual and other problems helped precipitate an annulment from his marriage with his first wife, when he was in his middle 30's, after a year-long marriage. This second therapeutic foray was also of short duration. Mr. T initially saw the doctor in individual sessions, but when the therapist suggested group therapy as well, the patient was unable to bring himself to expose his "failings" before a "public tribunal." Finally, when his second marriage (which he entered into shortly after the age of 50) also began to come apart because of his chronic sexual and characterological difficulties, he sought help with the man who ultimately referred him to me.

In the third treatment, the doctor (an analytically oriented psychotherapist) found Mr. T to be an introspective individual who was interested in understanding the historical determinants of his difficulties. Although the patient had achieved some intellectual insight into the roots of his severe castration anxiety, such as his recognition of the fear of a fantasied retaliation by his stern father, if he were to have a successful sexual relationship with a woman, little headway in resolving his difficulties had been made.

Mr. T was born and raised in a mixed ethnic neighborhood in a poor section of New York City. His parents' money concerns were a constant source of friction, and the message he received from his mother's diatribes against his father was that his father was not providing her with enough of anything—money, love, security, or sexual gratification. The father, enraged at the mother's polemics, would smash his clenched fists until they bled upon the kitchen table or bang his head against the wall. He neither raised his fists nor his voice directly against the mother, however. At the height of his fury, he would dramatically and ceremoniously spit into the kitchen sink, with a look of enormous contempt. The mother then would disgustedly cease her tirade. The patient, an only child, would look upon these scenes in silent horror and with the expectation that one day the father would explode and that he would either murder his wife or splatter his own brains upon the kitchen walls. The patient would then be left an orphan, alone and homeless. Neither parent seemed to realize or care about how their battles affected their only child.

The only escape from familial tensions was Mr. T's being peripherally included in the activities of a warm, loving Italian family who lived nearby. This family had three daughters. Two of the girls were a good deal older than the patient, and they and the mother of the family treated him cordially, an experience unknown in his own home. The third daughter, L, was a year younger than the patient, and from their earliest years, they felt a special warmth and friendship for each other. In their shared fantasies in childhood, they spoke of getting married when they grew up. He would make a great deal of money for her and she would have many children (both boys and girls) and their lives would be a series of tranquil days and nights, never marred by fights, and food and love would be heaped on everyone in great abundance. None of the difficulties that would later becloud their relationship ever entered into these fantasies and Mr. T's adoration for L and her family seemed to know no bounds.

In adolescence, the idyllic childhood companionship blossomed forth into a relatively mature type of love relationship. Whereas L's mother cast a benign eye upon their romance, L's father was not pleased with the idea of having a Jewish son-in-law. A religious man, he had thought of his youngest daughter's becoming a nun, perhaps even a nursing sister. He informed L of his wishes and instructed her at great length about the difficulties of a mixed marriage. She, however, countered his objections with her fantasies of true love conquering all, in the style of the protagonists of the play *Abie's Irish Rose*. Mr. T's parents, however, were of quite a different mind. They dramatically refused him permission to invite L to his bar mitzvah (his coming into manhood in the Jewish religion) and he embarrassed himself (and them) by having his voice crack during the chanting of the particular passages from the Torah. Following this misadventure, Mr. T's parents forbade him to ever bring L into their house again.

The patient continued to see L, however, and at 16, when he was walking hand-in-hand with her, they ran into his father on the street. The patient bowed his head in fear and could not bring himself to speak but L implored Mr. T's father to allow them to "keep steady company." His father acknowledged her presence by spitting on the sidewalk near her. The patient felt helpless to defend L or to oppose his father's rage. When he returned home later that day, he was given an ultimatum by his mother that he must stop seeing his "shiksa sveetheart" or he would be thrown out of the house.

Mr. T responded to this humiliating episode with anxiety attacks and somatic complaints (a dry throat, headaches, and stomach upsets). Although he continued to meet secretly with L for a number of months, he felt increasingly ashamed of himself in her presence and began to think of himself as inadequate. Although the two of them had never done anything more with each other sexually than to kiss and to pet lightly, Mr. T began to imagine then that he would be unable to perform sexually with L. He felt increasingly tortured by his doubts about himself and began to see her less and less frequently, finally breaking off the relationship when he was 17, when he entered one of the city colleges to study business. His life seemed empty without her (and without her warm family) and for several years he felt as if he were simply going through the motions at school and in his daytime jobs.

During the listless years he attended college, and for a number of years thereafter, Mr. T rarely dated, although women found him good looking and a few neighborhood girls even asked him to go out with them. When he did go out, he did not make any sexual advances toward the women, and his only sexual release came in his solitary, guilt-ridden masturbation. He fantasized himself with the prostitutes he saw walking on the streets and occasionally with one of the neighborhood girls who had a loose reputation. On the rare occasions L involuntarily crept into one of his fantasies, he would become violently ashamed of himself and would not allow himself to masturbate further.

In the initial jobs Mr. T held after graduating from college, he never seemed to measure up to the anticipation of his employers. They imagined that this "big, strapping young man" would be a "real go-getter," but this was not the case. Fired from one job after another, he came to share in the vitriol heaped upon his father's head by his mother. Neither of them seemed manly enough in her eyes, with respect to making money, and in the patient's mind, this resonated with his own indictments of himself for what he feared to be his sexual inadequacy.

When Mr. T attempted sexual intercourse with a prostitute, in his middle 20's, and was unable to achieve an erection, his worst fears seemed to have been realized. As if that were not enough, when he was 27 years old, he heard that L had married and moved away from the neighborhood. Once more, he responded with the same somatic symptoms (a dry throat, headaches, and stomach pains). Aware of a vague feeling of anger toward his parents, he was unable to verbalize any of his thoughts to them. The overriding feelings, however, were those of depression at L's loss and shame at not having been man enough to hold onto the one woman he loved.

Some months after L's marriage, Mr. T's mother launched into one of her typical tirades against her husband. With all the high-paying jobs available in the defense industry in the period prior to the entry of America into World War II, she was appalled that the father was still unable to support his wife properly. This diatribe proved to be the one that broke the camel's back. With a scream of fury and a bubble of spittle issuing from his lips, the father sprang toward the mother. Then suddenly, as the patient once more looked on in silent horror, his father fell, dead from a heart attack before he hit the floor.

The patient, terrified, suffered a renewed series of anxiety attacks and somatic symptoms. His mother showed no remorse for her contributions to her husband's demise and had no sympathy for her son's anxieties and depressive response to his father's death. She remarried after the usual year of mourning for her spouse had ended and informed her son that he must seek out new lodgings, as it would not be reasonable for him to be living with her and her new husband. The patient consented to this further rejection by his mother and quickly found a room in a boarding house. When the middle-aged female who ran the house (a woman slightly younger than his mother) attempted to seduce him one evening, and he was unable to achieve an erection, he fled with his few possessions and was never able to return. At this time, he had his first unsuccessful experience with psychotherapy.

Mr. T's life was altered considerably when he was drafted into the army during World War II and sent to Officers' Candidate School, where he successfully completed the course and became a second lieutenant in the Quartermaster Corps. Although he was not directly involved in combat, his unit came under fire on a number of occasions during the Italian campaign and for the first time in many years, he felt that he had survived a dangerous "performance type situation" during which his self-regard remained intact.

In the army, Mr. T was able to regard himself as a "man among men," and after the liberation of Rome, he had one of the few episodes of successful erection and ejaculation after intromission of his life, with a young Italian girl who attached herself to him and to the chocolate bars and nylon stockings he waved in her direction. It was only during the treatment with me, that he came to realize that this girl had borne a rather startling resemblance to his former sweetheart, L.

Following his separation from the army after World War II, Mr. T obtained a job in a business that utilized many of the skills he had learned in the service. For the first time, both financial success and repeated promotions in his job came his way, and he ultimately became a partner in the firm. As his career began to prosper, he began to date a Jewish girl considerably younger than he was. She had had little or no prior sexual experience. When Mr. T made few advances to her, she took it as a sign of his respect for her virginity. When the patient took her to meet his mother, who was dying from metastatic breast cancer, his mother suggested that he marry the girl. He embraced his mother and quickly followed her advice, although he realized that he did not really love his wife. His mother died shortly before the wedding was to have occurred, thus necessitating a brief delay in plans. Mr. T, surprised at how little emotion he was able to muster at the loss, briefly blamed himself for his lack of depth as a person.

On their wedding night and during a month-long honeymoon trip to Europe, Mr. T was unable to achieve an erection. He felt immense frustration and shame before his bride, who rather quickly began to recognize that what she had taken as a sign of respect was really a harbinger of a rather profound disturbance in her husband's sexual functioning. In this setting, Mr. T attempted to satisfy his wife by means of manual clitoral manipulation or by cunnilingus after his perfunctory attempts to achieve erection and intercourse would fail. Initially, his wife helped him obtain sexual release through manual masturbation, but this became less and less frequent, as she became increasingly disenchanted.

When the couple returned from the honeymoon, his wife asked Mr. T if he had ever had this problem with anyone else. He initially lied to her and told her that the difficulty was something new for him, inventing stories of potent escapades during his service career and earlier life. When he saw that this made his wife feel guilty, inadequate, and depressed over the next few months, he was sorry and told her that he had indeed experienced these difficulties in the past and had even consulted a psychiatrist for the treatment of the problems, without much benefit. His wife, unfortunately, responded with considerable anger at his revelations and berated him for having lied to her and tricking her into a sexless marriage. As he listened, he was reminded of his mother's tirades against his father. He vividly recollected his father's spitting into the sink, and the rageful sound when he died.

Mr. T then felt a momentary pain in his chest and feared that he, too, might die and wondered if this might not be the best solution for all concerned. Instead of dying, however, he merely slumped to the floor and began to cry. His wife was too angry to succor or comfort him for his acute psychological pain and humiliation. Shortly thereafter, she left him and returned to her parents' home. Although the couple attempted a brief reconciliation a month later, it was short lived and doomed to failure, by virtue of their mutual rage.

After separation from his first wife, and after proceedings for an annulment had been started, Mr. T again consulted a psychiatrist. He did not like or trust the doctor he was sent to, a man considerably older than he was. He felt that the doctor did not appreciate how painful some of the answers to the questions he was asking were to give. Although he agreed with the doctor's suggestion that he had a great deal of difficulty expressing anger, he saw little correlation between that and his sexual performance. When the therapist suggested that the patient might help his problem with aggressivity if he were to enter group therapy, Mr. T, feeling that he could not tolerate the humiliation, unilaterally terminated psychotherapy.

Over the next decade and one-half, Mr. T prospered further in his business career. He was known more for his tact in business negotiations and in the handling of his partners than for his aggressivity. His personal life was rather lonely. He maintained a few long-term friendships, but he could never bring himself to talk of his sexual difficulties with anyone. He entertained elegantly, maintained a lovely apartment, and traveled frequently, acquiring a considerable modicum of culture and polish that belied his humble origins. Perhaps his most surprising accomplishment was that he also became a consummate poker player. He was able to read his opponents' strategies perfectly, and knew just when and with whom to bluff and when to play the hand straight. He almost invariably won at cards and almost always would muse after an evening's play, "I'm lucky at cards and unlucky in love."

Sexually, his life consisted of secret, infrequent liaisons with secretaries or other lower-level employees of his firm. The long practiced pattern of satisfying the woman with manual manipulation of her clitoris or by cunnilingus would then be followed by occasional attempts at penetration, which would generally fail, with the episode culminating in his being masturbated to orgasm by the woman. On a few occasions, he was able to achieve a partial erection and partial penetration, and then he felt some real pleasure in the act. In the main, however, his sexual interactions with women were compulsive, with little real gratification.

At a surprise party thrown for him by a friend, Mr. T met the woman who was to become his second wife. A slightly older, attractive Jewish woman, she had been married several times previously and had several grown children by former spouses. As the two of them began to date, she emphasized the idea of wishing to find companionship for her waning years and deemphasized the idea of sexuality and romance, maintaining that such notions had gotten her into considerable difficulty in the past. She seemed quite supportive of the patient's obvious sexual problems and told him that they did not really matter that much to her. He was grateful to her for not making an issue of his performance problems; shortly thereafter he proposed marriage to her, and was accepted.

For the first few years of the marriage, both parties seemed rather happy with the arrangement they had worked out. Mr. T squired his wife to a never-ending round of parties and charity balls and the two of them traveled extensively. But beneath the surface veneer of good cheer and companionship, cracks were beginning to show in the foundations of the marriage. The second Mrs. T began to drink quite heavily at parties and would become subtly insulting of her husband, although she never singled out his sexual performance for her derisive comments.

When Mr. T would complain about her jibes, she would tell him that he was being hypersensitive and she would then proceed to drink herself to sleep. The one or two semi-successful sexual encounters the couple had experienced earlier in their marriage were not repeated after she began to criticize him in social situations. When his second wife attempted to goad Mr. T into fighting with a man who was talking suggestively to her at a dinner party, and then openly criticized him for his "lack of manliness" in having failed to defend her "honor," Mr. T became enraged and almost struck her. He left the party without her and soon separated from her and began divorce proceedings. He then began the treatment with the third therapist, who ultimately referred him to me.

When I first saw Mr. T and obtained fragments of the history I have presented thus far, I was ambivalent about psychoanalysis for him as the treatment of choice. Although he seemed in good health, which a note from his internist corroborated, I felt reluctant about beginning to work on what I felt would be a rather lengthy treatment with a man 59 years old. But even more than his age, I wondered about whether or not his long-standing potency problem could be modified at this late date. Although he had been married twice and had maintained a number of friendships, the quality of his object-relationships concerned me. The one with L had been a close one; in later years, there had been no friend close enough to reveal his sexual performance difficulties to. Also, his earlier pyschotherapy had not been successful.

A number of factors finally convinced me to attempt analysis. One of these was the very evident warmth that Mr. T communicated in his interviews with me. Although he gave a history of past secretiveness, he now projected a sense of openness and a ready facility to reveal unconscious material. This was especially evident to me in our third sitting-up session, when he revealed a dream he had had the night before in which he felt that his feet were "mired" in quicksand and his body was being dragged down to some nether world. As he cried out for help, a powerful arm reached out of the darkness and pulled him free. His associations immediately went to his wishes and expectations with respect to treatment with me. I finally confronted him with this apparent dichotomy between his current presentation in treatment with me and his past history of therapeutic failures. He acknowledged that my observation was probably accurate, as he had been more "closed up" in the past. "But now that I'm going to be 60," he said, "there isn't any more time to hold it all in. My father died when he was 60 and the only reason that he didn't live any longer was that he held his feelings all bundled up inside of him all of his life. I've done the same thing for most of mine. If I'm ever going to be happy, now's the time to open up and change things. I don't know if it's you or me, doc, but I feel freer with you than with my other therapists. Maybe it's both of us. Whatever it is, it certainly feels good."

I found this speech an impressive one, as it showed a strong motivational factor and a strong positive transference potential, which probably had not been present in his earlier therapies. His pronouncements also underscored his desire to achieve happiness, even at this late date in his life, and his desires to surpass his father. The presence of both wishes seemed to be rather positive determinants, as they indicated a mutability in his character structure I would not have expected from his history. Let me add one final determinant to the list of factors that influenced my decision to analyze Mr. T. He was a very likeable man, one with whom I could readily empathize. I wished to help him; I came to recognize that this wish had been stimulated by my desires to rescue my own father, who was nearing death at the time that I began to analyze Mr. T.

Mr. T was at ease with the idea of using the couch from the very beginning of the analysis. "It's a lot easier for me to say things to you in this way," he observed, "than by having to look you in the eye when I talk about them. I don't have to feel quite as judged this way. Intellectually, I know that it's my own judgments that I'm talking about, but when I'm looking at you, it certainly feels as if they're coming from you." It was only some months later, that I found out that another factor contributing to his initial high spirits about being on the couch, was his idea of having been selected by me as being a suitable candidate for analysis. He had researched the subject of treatment modalities among those friends of his who had undergone therapy or analysis, revealing to them only that he was thinking of seeking some form of treatment because of his continuing unhappiness since the breakup of his second marriage. He had been informed by some knowledgeable friends that analysis was a more intensive kind of treatment and that it generally probed more deeply into the past. He was also led to believe that not everyone was judged to be suitable for such a treatment method and that it was unlikely that he would be recommended for analysis at his age.

Given these data, when I did suggest analysis to him after six sessions of evaluation, he was elated, as if he had been chosen for an exclusive club. I might add here that, aside from the obvious narcissistic gratification of having been chosen for this "select" treatment, the very efforts involved in his research indicated even more of a motivation for change than I was privy to at the time I decided to analyze him.

During the early sessions on the couch, Mr. T interspersed his rather methodical rendition of his history with bits and pieces of information of his day-to-day life. As he was describing his past sexual "weaknesses" and "failures" to me, he was exhibiting his triumphs and successes in business and his ready familiarity with world travel and elegant wining and dining. Along with these references to both his idealized and devalued self-representations were fleeting remarks about how happy he was that he was in analysis with a "younger, vigorous man," someone who also seemed to be "gentle and unflappable." My being unflappable was defined by him as being equivalent to my being able to "tolerate" anything he might say without my being "hurt or angered by it."

When I commented to him on the projection of his own fears of being hurt or angered by things that I might say to him, he reported feeling tearful for a moment, as if it were the first time in his life that anyone had ever really understood his sensitivity, that "thin skin" of his that had been so easily bruised in the past. The idealization of me in Mr. T's answers to my initial comments was certainly an important aspect of the initial transference response. There were, however, hints of other transference responses in the material in the session on the couch in the early weeks of the analysis.

One of these became apparent toward the end of the first month of analysis, when Mr. T recalled the initial dream about being drawn down into the quicksand and the helping hand he had seen me as extending to him to help free him. "It's funny," he said, "I think I had that same dream again last night. Only this time it was very dark in the dream, as if the quicksand was almost black in color and I was deeply mired in it." He became silent and when I inquired as to his thoughts, he was reluctant to relate them. "I guess I better say what I was thinking of," he observed, "otherwise

I won't get anywhere in here with you. The black color of the quicksand reminds me of the color of your couch. Maybe everything's not quite so rosy as I thought it would be in here. I think I'm afraid of what's going to come out in the analysis. Maybe it's better to leave it all buried."

I observed to Mr. T that his comments on the dream seemed to refer to his need to play the ostrich and to bury his head as well as his feet in the (quick)sand, and to thereby continue to remain in the dark. I further related his wish to avoid going deeper in the analysis to his fears of what dark destruction might be wreaked on him by me during its course, since he had referred in the dream to being "mired" in quicksand, and my name is Myers. I felt a need, however, to temper my remarks, by pointing out that he had managed to overcome his reluctance to talk to me of his fears, which would help his future progress.

At the time, my reassurance type of response of reinforcing his efforts at overcoming his resistance to talk of his fears of the destructive potential of the analysis, seemed almost "intuitive." It was, however, a response that "diluted" the direct type of transference interpretation I would have normally made to a younger analytic patient. This "dilution factor" type of interpretation is similar to the kind that one might make to an adolescent who exhibits intense fears of being overwhelmed by his drive derivative wishes in the postpubertal period.

In retrospect, I have had many second thoughts about whether or not Mr. T required any of the "kid glove" treatment I occasionally utilized in my interpretations to him in the early phases of analysis. Despite his age, he really seemed as resilient to me as most younger patients, with respect to being able to "bear the brunt" of most directly stated transference interpretations. Hence, I wonder whether or not my "intuitive" response of "protecting" him from further narcissistic mortifications, which might have been incurred through more baldly stated interpretations of the transference, did not really stem from my own need to protect him from my own unconscious hostile wishes, probably once more stemming from my feelings toward my dying father.

As Mr. T began to talk about his day-to-day interactions with his partners and clients, it became evident that he was utilizing his skills at negotiation and diplomacy to avoid more direct, aggressively tinged confrontations with people. When I commented on this, he fell silent and then spoke of feeling criticized by me. I said nothing at this juncture, and he drifted off into other material until the end of the session.

When he returned the next day, he said: "You know, I felt a kind of challenge by what you said to me in here yesterday. I'm glad that you did that. No one's ever really cared enough about me to goad me into acting like a man, without cutting the bottom out from under me at the same time. I think that my initial feeling of being criticized was my old "thin skin" showing through again. It was only after the session had ended that I realized that that wasn't what you really meant to convey by your comment. You really had my best interests at heart and were trying to encourage me to act more manly. I got the feeling that you really want me to succeed and I'm grateful to you for that. Even with L, she did the talking for me that time with my father. But here with you in the analysis, you want me to do all the talking for myself. You want me to be the man!"

In essence, it was apparent from the patient's monologue that he not only saw me as an idealized parental imago, but that he also regarded me as a more loving superego figure than any he had dealt with in his past. This depiction of me as a loving, encouraging superego figure was a very prominent feature of the positive transference relationship to me throughout much of the analysis. This is not to say that I did not encounter many responses in which I was also seen as a stern, prohibiting, and judgmental parental figure. Rather, it is to state that the predominant response to me was one in which I was seen as a benign superego representative, rather than a malignant one. Hence, a positive, mutative (Strachey, 1934) effect was more often conferred upon my interpretations than was a negative, destructive one. What puzzled me for a long time was the reason for this positive response. Mr. T had never felt especially good about any of his past therapists. Why should he be so positively inclined toward me? The answers to my question were only to be revealed over a period of many months.

In one session toward the end of the first year of the analysis, Mr. T spoke of the great enjoyment and satisfaction he had experienced in seeing a Western in which a younger gunfighter had helped an aging sheriff rid a town of a band of desperadoes. He noted how the actor who played the gunfighter was blond and superficially resembled me. "But it's more than that," he said, "more than just wanting you to help me be a man. It's what I think that I wanted to be able to do with my own father. To make him into a man so that he could stand up to my mother, instead of just spitting into that goddam sink. If he'd've been a man, it'd've been so much easier for me to be one, too. I'd've had his tacit permission. That's one of the most important things I feel in here with you. The permission for me to be a man."

In the rest of that session, we went on to concentrate on the dangers both he and his father had perceived in allowing themselves to be aggressive men. I was struck, however, by the feeling that Mr. T was somehow borrowing from my "youth," to undo, in fantasy, the negative identification with the castrated male figure, his father. This identification had been formed when he repeatedly witnessed his parents' fights during his childhood and adolescence. I further realized that one of the facets of his personality that made it easier for me to deal with him was his relative lack of envy. He did not wish to "steal" my youth from me. Rather, he wished to "borrow" it, so that he might learn how to develop his own sense of manliness, and then he could simply return it. I only imparted some of these thoughts to him at a later date when he revealed similar wishes for me to aid him in his quest for manliness. This occurred in the setting of his relating a dream to me, in which a young boy helped him work his way through a dangerous maze to freedom. The maze was in a prison guarded by vicious jailors, some of them women.

"I think you're right," he said. "It isn't just a question of having loved my father at some level, though I think that I did. It's more a question of his being the only game in town. He was the only man I had around me to protect me from my mother. She could be such a vicious bitch, the way she cut him down so often, about his not making enough money. I always felt as if she were cutting me down, too. . . . I guess that my feelings of doubt about myself as a man must have started a long time before the incident with L during my adolescence." Although the dangerous maze made me think of the black quicksand of the earlier dream, and both might be seen as relating to his fears of the woman (his mother) and her dangerous vagina, I only commented at that time upon his transference wishes for me to aid him by lending him my "vigorous youth," as he had wished to lend his "strength and manliness" to his father, so that the two of them might then overcome the dangerous, emasculating mother.

"You're so right. Maybe if I could've helped him withstand her vicious onslaughts, he might've still been alive today." Mr. T cried after this realization, as if he were finally being allowed to mourn for his father and to set his guilt (and shame) to rest over his own inadequate attempts to save his father from the deadly jibes of the harpy mother. It might be worthwhile to mention here that such comments as this from the patient made me feel warmly disposed toward him, as my own father had just recently died at that time and Mr. T's rescue wishes toward his father quite clearly resonated with my own toward mine. Fortunately, I was able to see the basis of this countertransference response and it did not interfere in my handling of my relationship with him.

Another aspect of Mr. T's positive feelings toward me also emerged from his associations to the dream about the maze. "You know," he said, "it may sound crazy . . . but ever since I first saw you, I've had the feeling that the two of us have quite a resemblance to each other physically. We could almost be father and son." He remained silent for some moments and then added: "If you were really my son, like the young boy helping me in the dream, it'd mean that I really had been a successful man in my life and a potent one. Maybe the resemblance is just a wish, doc, but I still feel that you look a lot like me. You could do worse, you know I'm not a bad-looking guy." Either way, as idealized father or as idealized son, I was seen as bolstering his own sense of himself as a man, thereby undoing the narcissistic traumata in his past and allowing him to mourn his missing manliness.

During the middle of the second year of the analysis, Mr. T became embroiled in some business proceedings involving the purchase of his firm by another, larger one. As the principals for the other corporation became more and more aggressive during the negotiations, the patient began to shed some of his customary gentleness and diplomacy and became quite outspoken in countering their demands. When the deal was finally closed, the management of the organization that had purchased Mr. T's firm expressed their admiration for his newfound aggressivity by rewarding him with a high level executive position in the new company and a seat on the board of directors. He was thrilled that he had been able to stand up to the "tough men" on the other side and attributed his success to the analysis and to the strength I had "infused" into him. Although there was some truth in his statement, I felt it incumbent on me to try to confront the continuing idealization of me and of the analytic process, as it was obvious that this idealization allowed much important material to be screened out of his treatment.

"What do you mean by the strength which I've been able to infuse into you?," I asked.

"I don't know," he answered. "It's pretty much like what I've been saying here all along. I have the feeling of borrowing something from you, your vigor, for want of a better word."

In reply, I noted that we both understood a great deal about that aspect of what he had been speaking of, but my question right then centered on his use of the word "infusion." He was silent and when he began to speak again, his general good humor of a few moments before was subdued.

"I guess it's comparable to an intravenous drip in a hospital, where the doctor gives the patient something to nourish and sustain him. When you 'needle' me in a nice way into acting more aggressively, it's like you're injecting some of the essence of your own manliness into me, or as we used to say in the army, some of your own spit and vinegar."

We were both struck by the words of his last phrase, and it hardly needed my repetition of them to get him to associate to them.

"My father's spitting in the sink," Mr. T observed, "was the only evidence of his masculinity, when it came to his standing up to my mother. It must have meant something to her, too. It must have scared her, because she'd shut up when he'd do that. Only that last time he spit at her, it cost him his life. It's funny that I say that, because I know that that's not literally true. Yet somehow I think that I must still believe it to be true at some kind of a feeling level."

After a moment's silence, I commented to the patient that in his mind, spitting certainly seemed to be dangerous, to other people or to oneself. I further noted that from what he had just intimated, it must be a particularly dangerous thing to do when you directed your spit at a woman with whom you were involved. He seemed stunned and shaken by my comments, as if I had suddenly withdrawn the helping hand that had sustained him and dropped him into the dark quicksand of his initial dream.

"I never thought of that connection before," and then he lapsed into an icy, withdrawn silence that continued until the end of the session.

Mr. T. arrived a quarter of an hour late for his next session, something that had not happened in his prior year and one-half of analysis. He spoke of important duties connected with his new job that had made it necessary for him to be late, duties that might regularly interfere with his ability to keep all his future appointments with me. Then he lapsed into silence once more. After a few moments of this, I said that I thought that he must have been very angry with me because of what I had said to him the day before.

"I still am," he exploded. "I thought that you were on my side and you turn out to be just like everyone else. When I'm feeling high, you cut the bottom out from under me with your typical analytic preoccupations with sex. I thought you were different than my other therapists, but now I'm not so sure anymore."

Although his allusion to feeling high and then having the bottom cut out from under him was not lost on me (nor on him), I felt it important at this point to let him pursue his first real expression of anger toward me and toward the analytic process. I thus remained silent.

"You're just like my mother," he said. "You're never satisfied with anything. No matter what I do, no matter how well I perform, it's never enough for you, just as nothing that my father or I could do was ever enough for her."

As he spoke, Mr. T's voice became increasingly harsh and strained, and then barely loud for me to hear. When I asked him to repeat one of his sentences, he whispered: "My throat is very dry, it's hard for me to talk now."

I commented then: "When you get angry with someone, as you are with me right now, the 'spit' must dry right up in your throat, so you can't quite let them know just how you really feel."

Mr. T interrupted and said: "Like the time at my bar mitzvah when my voice cracked. Or when I got the dry throats when L begged my father to let us keep company. Or the time when she got married. Dammit, I still feel mad at you for being such a killjoy yesterday, but I know now that you were right in what you were saying. I do dry up when I get angry. I must be afraid of killing them or maybe myself with my spit, just like my father was. You're probably right with the connection between spitting and sex, too. Maybe I do think that my sperm is like spit, they both begin with the same letters. Maybe I feel it's just as deadly."

I said that I was sure that he did feel that way about injecting and "infusing" his sperm into a woman. And if he did feel that way about his sperm, since his penis was the organ that fired the deadly spit–sperm into the woman, it must be essential for him to always keep his gun "uncocked," lest he damage or kill the woman or be killed by her. Much of the time in the next year and one-half of the analysis was spent working through the material and the interpretations that arose in these two important sessions and as a direct result of them.

Although Mr. T's daily utterances continued to contain a goodly number of allusions to his work, in particular to examples of his increasingly aggressive performance on his job, more of our time was spent dealing more directly with his sexual performance problems. He felt shame at revealing his masturbatory practices to me, especially when he had to lay bare the performance difficulties that permeated even his private fantasies.

In the main, in Mr. T's masturbatory fantasies, as in his real-life sexual experiences with his secretary and with other employees, he concentrated on satisfying the woman orally and manually. Only rarely did the primary focus of such fantasies (or of his real life sexual experiences) center on his own sensual or sexual gratification. Although he might allow himself in reality (or imagine himself in fantasy) to be masturbated to orgasm, he felt little real pleasure in his climax, as he was so suffused with feelings of shame and guilt at being in such a passive, ineffectual, impotent posture vis-à-vis the woman. As the third year of the analysis ended, he became convinced of the veracity of the earlier interpretation of his fears of killing the woman (or of being harmed or killed himself by her) during sexual intercourse. Although he began to attempt penetration somewhat more frequently with his paramours, his success rate in these attempts was still quite low.

During a session in the middle of the fourth year of the analysis, Mr. T informed me that he had had a frightening dream the night before. "I dreamt that I was in Brazil on business and one of my associates suggested that we take a sightseeing plane and fly over to look at the Amazon River. As the plane flew low over the river, it looked very dark and ominous to me and I saw some alligators slithering by on the river banks. Suddenly the engine began to sputter in the plane and we began to lose altitude. We were obviously going to crash into the river. Just as we started to hit the water, I saw one of the alligators open its jaws and flash its rows of teeth at me. I felt a kind of primordial terror come over me and then I woke up."

In his associations to the dream, Mr. T linked the dark, ominous river with the frightening quicksand of his first dream in the analysis. On a number of occasions in the past, when the quicksand dream had come to mind, we had been able to connect his fears of being drawn into the quicksand and being unable to get out with his fears of a similar disaster befalling him if he tarried too long inside a woman's vagina. This time, we were able to add another feature to those involved in his fears concerning the vagina.

"Those teeth," he said, "they scared the hell out of me. I could just imagine them biting my legs off." "Or perhaps your penis," I added. "I think you're right," he concurred. "I must be afraid of something terrible like that happening to me inside of a woman. My God, an Amazon, no less." He was silent for a moment and then he continued: "It's funny, I did something different last night. I slept with S (his secretary) and instead of sending her home in a cab after it was over, I let her spend the night with me. I'm not sure if I've ever done that before with a woman I wasn't married to. It's not that I really care anymore about S than I did before, but I didn't have that feeling of anger that I usually have with a woman when the sex is over."

I suggested to the patient then that as his anger toward women was diminishing, his wishes for sexual and emotional closeness might be increasing, and that these wishes might arouse the anxiety expressed in his fears of the dangerous vagina (dentata). When he began to move on to other material, I brought his attention back to the dream and inquired as to what his associations were concerning Brazil and possibly the river.

"I don't really have any thoughts about either of them," he said. "I've certainly never considered doing any business down there. I remember once seeing a film, a kind of marvelous travelogue through South America, in which they were driving a herd of cattle across a river there, possibly the Amazon. They let one of the cows go in first, as a sacrifice to the pirranhas in the river, and while the fish were eating that one cow down to the very bone, the gauchos drove the rest of the herd safely across the river."

I observed that he had once more described an image involving being eaten down to the "bone" by the deadly teeth of the pirranhas in the dark river, a further corroboration of the alligator in the vagina fear he had spoken of a short while before.

"You're right," he said, and then paused. "Maybe this is pretty far out," he continued, "but my mother's first name starts with the letters B and A. I'm probably just stretching things there. Maybe I should get back on safer ground."

In response to these latter comments, I said: "Perhaps you're saying that it's always safer when you don't let things get stretched, or allow yourself or your penis to fly too high. As you've said before, when you used to try to show off to your mother, she'd always cut the ground out from underneath your feet."

Mr. T pondered the meaning of my remarks, and then asked, "Do you really think that I wanted her sexually? My mother, I mean?" When I said nothing, he went on with his own thoughts. "It sounds so damn textbooky, to want to have sex with your own mother. I thought I was supposed to fear my father's chopping off my balls for wanting that, not my mother's doing it."

I noted that he certainly had been afraid of his father, as when he had been too fearful to defend L against him. But he had also been fearful of being harmed by his mother.

"That's true. What you said before, about my wanting more closeness with women now, it must be true. I'm getting older and I want to have it before I die. Maybe the dark river is death, too. My wanting closeness isn't something new, you know. I've always really dreamed about that. Whenever I'd try to hug my mother or to snuggle up to her as a child, she'd push me away. Besides hating her for that, I must have felt incredibly rejected by her, pretty much the way my father must have felt with her. He wasn't the warmest guy in the world by any means, but whatever warmth and love I got from either of them came from him. That's why I became so close to L and to her family. I used to spend hours daydreaming about being a member of their family. I knew her father really wanted a son and I wanted to fulfill that wish of his, so that he would love me, too. God, I wanted to be loved so badly by someone. Why couldn't she see that? Why couldn't my mother have given me the slightest iota of it? Damn her. . . . Why did I ever let L get away? She was the only one who ever really did love me."

With these pronouncements, Mr. T began to cry in a manner in which he had never really cried before during the analysis. He continued to sob this way until the end of the session, tearfully mourning the loss of L, bemoaning his rejection by his mother, and expressing his fears of never achieving closeness to a woman before his death.

In the weeks and months that followed, Mr. T continued to reflect upon his longings for closeness with a woman. As the summer vacation separation approached, he spent sessions crying bitterly about his impending "loss" of me and about his fears of his own death. He was able to verbalize clearly for the first time in the analysis his rage to me over his dependency upon me and his need for me to sustain his life and we were able to link this with his earlier feelings toward his mother and toward L. Despite the intensity of his anger, anxiety, and sadness before my vacation, he was able to wish me well when I left. I might add here, that none of the somatic symptoms that had plagued him during his adolescence troubled him at this stage of the analysis.

When he returned in the fall, he informed me that he had met a woman at a seaside resort who reminded him a great deal of L. The only difference was that this new woman, A, was blonde. She, too, was Italian, as L had been, and she seemed to have the same warmth as his childhood sweetheart. Although he had wined and dined her in great style, he had not attempted anything sexually with her.

"I guess that I was waiting for you to come back, doc, before I tried anything. I need my daily vitamin infusion from you, so that I can function. Besides, since we've always characterized anyone I've known who's been blonde as being a substitute for you, maybe all she is is your summer replacement."

I commented that perhaps she had been a replacement for both me and for L. He had, after all, been mourning our losses before I had left on vacation. What we really had to see, however, was whether or not he was able to perceive her as a separate individual, independent of either one of us.

The first weekend after my return from vacation, Mr. T took A with him on Saturday morning to his country home. It was still warm and they were able to spend the day swimming and playing tennis. At night, when they went to bed, he felt anxious as they snuggled together beneath the covers. For the first time in his life, however, he decided to reveal some of his anxieties to a woman in advance of any attempted sexual encounter.

"I've had a lot of problems all of my life," he blurted out, "sexually, I mean. Either I don't get hard or I come too quickly." A's response was to press him closer to her as if to assure him that things would work out in time. His voice broke momentarily, as he struggled to respond verbally to her non-verbal communication. His sobs, which had filled so many of our recent sessions, rose in his throat, but he was able to push them back and to blurt out: "Thank you. Thank you for being so kind. I really appreciate it."

Neither that night nor the next one, was Mr. T able to achieve an erection with A. But it felt good, nonetheless, he informed me on the following Monday, just to hold her close to him and to be held by her, in turn. He asked her whether or not he was frustrating her, and he offered to try to satisfy her in the accustomed ways (orally and manually). She replied that she preferred to wait for him to enter her. Yes, she wanted him, she had said, but she could and would wait. There was plenty of time.

Over the next few weeks, the two spent a great deal of time together, both during the week and on weekends. Mr. T felt a great deal of pressure to have an erection for A, but he was unable to. He wondered with me if telling her about being in treatment might be of any help to him in this regard. I inquired as to what his thoughts were about this matter.

"I think it's more of a way for me to really open up to her about my past. To tell her about my parents and about L and about my past failures." He was silent for a moment and then he asked: "Do you think I'm introducing this in order to offer excuses for myself?" Again I let him proceed with answering his own question. "I think I am in some way. Maybe I shouldn't do it."

At this juncture, I noted that whether he informed her of his being in analysis was his decision, but I wondered if one important facet of his desire to tell her might not have to do with his wish to more directly introduce me in some manner into the bedroom scene, perhaps as for security or to bolster his flagging sense of masculinity. Suffice it to say, I had long since stopped using the "kid glove" dilution factor type of transference interpretations with Mr. T.

"Would you object if I did use you that way?" he asked. And then in response to his own question, he answered: "No, I guess you really wouldn't."

The next night that he spent with A, he told her he was in analysis and he was pleased to hear her say that she, too, had been in therapy and that it had helped her a great deal after the death of her husband. He spoke to her about his parents and about his relationship with L in the past and even about his successful sex with the young Italian girl after the liberation of Rome.

"I'm glad that you have a thing for Italian women," she said. "Otherwise I'd feel left out. And I don't want to feel that way with you. I like you too much for that."

After their discussion that night, he managed a partial erection and was able to penetrate briefly before he ejaculated. Although it was not the perfect response he had hoped for, in fantasy, he was sufficiently elated with the result to come in beaming from ear to ear for the next session with me.

"You're a pretty powerful aphrodisiac, doc. All I have to do is think about you and I get an erection with A. You ought to market yourself, you'd make a fortune."

When I questioned him about his referring to me as the aphrodisiac he had utilized in order to help him, he snapped back: "There you go again, never letting anything go by. I know you're not trying to cut me down, as my mother did, but at moments like this, it sure feels that way. What am I supposed to tell you now? That it's really you I was fucking and not A? It's just not true!"

The broad smile vanished, and the anger that replaced it had also gone, to be replaced in turn by a sense of sadness and longing. "All I want to do is to be a man with her. I don't care whether I can accomplish that because of my homosexual wishes toward you or because of any other unconscious quirk in my makeup. I just want to accomplish it before I die."

I said to him that, at this time, it seemed as if he was very frightened of his success, not only as a man with A, but in allowing himself to be separate from me. I further observed that perhaps as important as the homosexual desires directed toward me, evident in his mental utilization of my image during the sexual act with A, was his continuing need to feel that he could not function as a separate person without my loving presence. Death was not only the unconscious punishment he perceived as resulting from being a successful (potent) man, it was also equated with his being a successfully separate person. Once more he cried at my comments, but his sense of sadness and longing had all but disappeared.

From that time on, Mr. T began to function with a much greater degree of success in his sexual relations with A. I cannot say that he ever achieved complete erectile potency on a regular basis, but both he and A were satisfied enough with the results to marry. Midway through the sixth year of the analysis, we agreed to terminate by the next summer. In the remaining months, there was a brief return of the potency difficulties, which we both related to his feelings concerning the end of the treatment and my impending loss. This passed, however, and the patient seemed genuinely happy with his new wife. We spoke of the future and of his plans after retirement and he expressed his wish to travel extensively with A and to show her the places he had come to love on his sojourns around the world. After receiving my assurance that he could return if and when he wished to, he threw his arms around me and gave me a bear hug and with mutual verbalizations of good wishes, he left my office.

In the Christmas cards that came for some years after his termination, I obtained some follow-up. He spoke of how much he was enjoying his life with A and also spoke of being asked to remain on at his job with the company after the usual retirement age because of their reluctance to lose him. All in all, it seemed a very happy result. Unfortunately, Mr. T died about five years after the termination of the analysis, shortly after his 70th birthday. His wife called and came in to see me. She said that he had often spoken of the analysis as the most important thing, next to their marriage, in his life. The "infusion" of my youth had not protected him from death, but it had allowed him to live out his last decade as a happier man.

At this juncture, let me underscore some of the more important features of Mr. T's case. A symptom of very long-standing duration, his potency problem, was resolved to a very considerable degree in a man who was in his middle 60's by the end of the six-year analysis. Such a salutory result proves the resiliency of the ego in many older patients and is evidence of their amenability to both psychoanalysis and psychoanalytically oriented psychotherapy. Although such salutory results in people of this age may not always be the rule, we should not be deterred from seeking out, in our consultative evaluations, just those individuals who will exhibit the degree of ego and superego flexibility to bring about the changes described in Mr. T. The factors involved in such assessments are not always easy ones to detail, although I shall delineate some of them in chapter 8.

Another cluster of features of Mr. T's case include the ready accessibility of unconscious material and the patient's capacity to recover childhood memories. In addition, he demonstrated an ease in free association and an ability to work with dream and fantasy material. As a consequence of these factors, he was able to form a pronounced transference neurosis, which he then was able to analyze to its genetic roots.

A third finding of importance in Mr. T's case was the profound boost to his motivation for therapeutic change that his age (and his wish for more happiness and longevity than his father had had) conferred upon him. His change in motivation and the evident thickening of his "thin skin" (his capacity for suffering narcissistic wounds as a result of therapeutic exposures and interpretations) both contributed to the ultimate success of the analysis. It seems highly unlikely that Mr. T developed a remarkably greater capacity for object-relationships during his analysis. Rather, it would be more accurate to state that the blunting of his original ability to relate in a warm intimate manner with individuals such as L and her family, was largely undone by the trust he developed with me in the transference relationship.

3

THERAPY OF AN ALCOHOLIC WOMAN:
Mrs. N

Mrs. N, a slightly overweight, though attractive, 54-year-old widow, was referred to me by her internist, who had been treating her with tranquilizers and antidepressants without any discernible benefit. She had confided to him that her usual drinking pattern had changed "over the past few years" and she was fearful that she was "on the verge of becoming an alcoholic."

Since the patient was a very articulate woman, she quickly verbalized the cogent observation that she was most apt to drink in social situations, particularly at those gatherings in which she saw herself as the "least successful" person present. Though she was a bit vague regarding the phrase "least successful," she consistently included the ideas of being "with someone" and "feeling lovable" as part of her definition.

Solitary drinking, or drinking to overcome trouble falling asleep, had not been a prominent part of Mrs. N's alcohol pattern until the few weeks prior to her seeing me. What had become a problem, however, was that if she had begun to drink excessively when she was with people, she would continue her drinking at home until she passed out. After such episodes, she would suffer from blackouts, and these memory lapses had frightened her into telling her internist about her drinking.

When I questioned her about feeling depressed or about suffering from any of the vegetative signs of depression, she denied these. "I don't really feel depressed," she said. "I think that I have a pretty good idea of what it looks like. I've seen a couple of friends of mine go through them at the menopause. That's not really what I'm feeling right now." Mrs. N had, incidentally, undergone a surgically induced menopause some ten years earlier, because of an advanced case of endometriosis. Seven years after her hysterectomy, her husband had died of a second heart attack. "My real problem is that I feel like a zero, a five-oh-plus zero," she announced. "I can't see what I've accomplished in my life. I don't mean to sound maudlin or melodramatic about it. And I'm not going to run out and shoot myself or gobble down a bunch of pills, though I suppose that you could say that my drinking amounts to the same damn thing. What I'm getting at, is that I can't see the point of it all.

"I'm an aging suburban housewife, with no kids [her only son had been killed in Vietnam when she was 49], no husband, a worthless degree in Art History, and no one out there to love me. I don't even have elderly parents who depend on me, so that I could resent taking care of them. I have absolutely no material impact on a living soul. It's so lonely out there, I could die. And then, when I even lose my own perception of myself, when I black out after drinking too much, that's just too damn much. It's like looking in the mirror and not seeing any image staring back at you. Just a bunch of glassy-eyed empty space. It's scary as hell!"

Mrs. N was the youngest of three children in a "typical WASP family" in one of the more "charming" Connecticut suburban towns an hour from New York City. Her mother, a transplanted southern belle, attempted to become interested in such local pursuits as gardening, tennis, and sailing, but soon "gave up the ghost" and settled down to the "serious drinking" that had characterized her forbears' existence south of the Mason-Dixon line. Her alcoholism was a "terrible cross for my brothers and I to bear," Mrs. N noted, in describing her mother, "she was so unpredictable. Some days'd be good and she'd cook up a storm. We'd be swimming in baked ham and sweet potatoes. Other days'd be lousy as hell. She'd hole up in her room and drink all day and the place'd smell of pee and puke by the time we got home from school and daddy'd get home from work. It was horrible. You never could invite anyone over after school because you'd never know whether it was going to be a good day or a bad one. I hated her for that quality, and so did my brothers."

The patient's father was described as the prototypical commuter. He rose to an executive position of considerable importance in one of the major advertising agencies in New York, more through his facility in avoiding internecine squabbles within the company and his sagacity in remaining with the agency through thick and thin, than through leap-frogging to other jobs in other agencies, as so many of his colleagues had done. But he was clearly a limited man, who preferred to "drive the ball a mile on the golf course" and to "come about in the wind" in his sailboat, rather than to come upon the solution to a client's problems or to puzzle out the complexities of agency life. The only aspect of his accounts that he seemed to truly enjoy was the social one. It certainly was more desirable, Mrs. N presumed, for her father to wine and dine his clients in the "elegant bistros of New York, than to return to his spouse, the dipso southern belle too soused to answer the doorbell for round seven, the time he'd normally be home if he came straight back from the office." The sadness underlying Mrs. N's clever patter was quite obvious, with the patter clearly being a long-term defense that had served her in good stead.

As the bits and pieces of the interaction between Mrs. N's parents emerged, it became apparent that there was a good deal of unspoken friction between them. Although they rarely fought openly, the patient always felt that her father was fantasizing about blasting her skull open when he would drive his "goddam golfballs" down the fairway at the country club. "They barely spoke to each other. They were like the proverbial two ships passing each other in the night. He'd work late most nights during the week and then spend the weekend at the club. By the time I was fourteen, she was drunk damn near all the time. Even though I was afraid I'd be more lonely than ever, I was glad when they decided to send me off to boarding school. I couldn't stand it at home anymore, with either one of them. He was no better than she was, really. He wasn't there for any of us then, either. I think he cared more then for the people who crewed for him sailing than he did for any of us. I don't understand why he never divorced her. Maybe he was just old fashioned, in that way. I don't even think he ever played around in all those nights out in New York. He was a strange man!"

Mrs. N's brothers were four and eight years older than she was. The elder was described in terms quite similar to those used by the patient in depicting her father. He, too, was caught up with sports, in a pathetic attempt to wring whatever modicum of attention he could from his father. When he went off to boarding school, he rather quickly became a problem drinker and by the time he managed to scrape through the Ivy League college his father had attended, he was a confirmed alcoholic. It was the patient who finally got across the severity of her brother's problem to her father, after the brother had appeared naked at the door of her room and collapsed on her carpet in a pool of his own urine.

The brother was summarily trundled off to the same drying-out establishments the mother had been sent to, with much the same lack of effect. Mrs. N's attempts to get her father to take any continuing interest in his elder son, fell on deaf ears, however, and the brother quickly rivaled his mother in the sheer quantity of alcohol he could consume. His brief, vainglorious career as a drinker ended abruptly one wintry evening (during the patient's sophomore year at boarding school) when he crashed his car through a guardrail on a highway overlooking the ocean. The patient cried bitterly at the brother's funeral, more in anger at her parents than for any real sense of loss for her brother.

In speaking of her four-year-older brother, she seemed a bit reluctant to describe him. When I asked her why, she said: "I don't really know him anymore. I thought I did when we were kids, but I think that was just an illusion. He was the closest person to me in the whole household and the closest person to my other brother, too. He was really a lovable, happy guy when we were kids, always clowning. He could even make my father and mother laugh, and that wasn't always easy to do. Then he met a girl, when he was in college, and fell head over heels in love with her. Only fate kept on dealing him cards from the bottom of the deck. She always managed to go to bed with his best buddy or something sweet like that. He thought he'd put an end to that by marrying her, but it didn't really change anything. Finally, she ran off with the guy who lived next door, or down the block anyway, and my brother never really got over it. Oh he's worked at different jobs and all that, and he still does. He even tried getting married again, but it was dead before it ever even got off the ground. And then he just sort of shriveled up into himself. The sweet kid who joked and wisecracked was gone and only a shell remained. Jesus, it makes me sad to think of him now. He's the only one of the three of us who doesn't drink, but for all that it matters in his life, he might as well. We still get together once in a while, but we don't have very much to say to each other anymore. It's funny, though, I never drink when I'm around him. It's as if that'd be the straw that broke the camel's back and I don't want to hurt him anymore than he's already been hurt. Maybe that's a sign of love. I don't know. I'm not sure I'm still capable of feeling such high-blown emotions."

The years in boarding school had not proven to be as lonely as Mrs. N had envisioned. Despite her outward antipathy toward her father, she too, had "inherited" her father's and older brother's aptitude for athletics. She became captain of the field hockey team in her junior year and of the tennis team in her senior year. Had her father shown more enthusiasm for her string of singles victories in tennis during her college career and in the years directly after her graduation, she might have risen beyond the level of the lower echelon championships she attained in the eastern circuit and gone on to climb the heights at Forest Hills and Wimbledon. He rarely even came to see her play, however, so her star never rose.

"Maybe it's just as well. I'm not even sure half the time that I really like the game anymore. I still play, you know, when I'm not hung over. I'm only a shadow of what I used to be, but once in a while it still all comes together for me. Then I feel like I've found a piece of myself, part of that image I spoke of that got lost in the mirror. Only it doesn't last for all that long, the feeling, and I have to climb back down off that high and see the empty shell staring back at me again. Depressing as that sounds, it still gives me pleasure when I whip an ace in or zing it to them with a crosscourt passing shot. God, I really am a chip off the old block. When I listen to myself talk in here, it's like hearing a reprise of my father going on about his golf game. I guess none of the apples in our family fell too far from the tree. Only shame was, that they all turned out to be so damned rotten."

Once she finished playing tennis, she gravitated to New York City where she worked in an art gallery. In the midst of what might have turned out to be the most important sale of her budding career, she was interrupted by a call from her father informing her of a turn for the worse in her mother's illness. What Mrs. N had passed off in her mother as an acute case of "whiskey fat" or "belleverdupois," in her usual joking manner, had turned out to be advanced cirrhosis of the liver with ascites. As the patient drove at breakneck speed to Connecticut, her mother was dying. By the time Mrs. N reached home, her mother was dead.

"I never even got to make a pass at saying goodbye to her, let alone telling her that I loved her, if I ever did. I was never there when anyone died. Neither my older brother, nor my father, nor my son. Not even my husband. I went down to the cafeteria to get a goddam cup of coffee and his heart went into a bloody arrhythmia and he was dead before I could get the second spoon of sugar into it. I have this horrible feeling that my punishment will be to die all by myself, with nobody else around me to even hold my hand."

After her mother's death, she left the city and returned to live in the family home in Connecticut. She kept house and prepared the meals for her father and he began to come home for dinner more regularly. "It wasn't as if we talked or anything. It was just that I felt closer to him, with my mother and brother dead. He'd come home at night and thank me for cooking a good dinner. I can't tell you how much that simple statement meant to me. It was practically the first compliment he'd ever paid me in my life.

"Once in a while, my father would ask me if I wanted to sail with him on the weekend. When I look back at it now, I think I'd've given my right arm to have gone out with him regularly in the boat. It wasn't the sailing, I really could care less about that. It was just the being asked. As if he were acknowledging me in some manner that he'd never even bothered to do so before. I went with him once or twice, but mostly I'd pretend that I had things to do and he'd mumble O.K., or something like that. Maybe that's what he really wanted me to do, to refuse to go out too often. Maybe he'd've been too embarrassed if I'd've been his regular 'sparring partner' on the boat. Too much intimacy with his daughter might've killed him even sooner than he actually died. I'll never know the answers to that now.

"The day after my 26th birthday, they called me from the club to say that he was dead. Within a year, I'd lost them both. He'd had a stroke during a race and was dead by the time they got him back to the dock. He'd've probably been mad as the dickens, if it'd've been someone else dying like that, not giving him a chance to finish the race and win the cup, or something. But I cried like hell when we buried him. I always seem to cry a lot at funerals, though I'm never sure of exactly for whom or what I'm crying."

Following her father's death, one of the young men who had crewed for him on his boat began to pay a good deal of attention to the orphaned daughter of his former skipper. Although she had dated a number of men at college and on the tennis circuit, and had even been "daring" enough to have slept with one or two men in her brief sojourn in New York City, she had never really felt close to any man outside of her next older brother. She had been "proposed to" by more than her share of eligible bachelors, but none of them had seemed to be the "right man" and she had turned them all down. After a time, the proposals had stopped and when she settled into managing the house for her father, it appeared for a while as if she might end up a spinster. These thoughts turned out to be idle speculation after Mr. N appeared. The unspoken communication between the two was that they had both lost a father in the skipper, as Mr. N, too, was an orphan. In all the years of their marriage, they never concretely verbalized that idea, but it was the unspoken bond that joined their lives together in the closest relationship that either of them had ever known.

Mr. N had entered his family's manufacturing business after his return from World War II. When his own father died, he turned what had been a rather small enterprise into a thriving success. He, too, had dated a good deal, but none of the women he had spent time with had meant anything to him before he met the patient. He quickly apprised her of his feelings for her, and when she responded to his confession in a like manner, they threw caution to the winds and were married. Three days after her 29th birthday (1950), their only son was born.

The new parents doted on their young son, in a manner that became more pronounced as each passing year and miscarriage increased their certainty that he was to be their only child. He was their golden-haired boy, but when he dropped out of college after his freshman year and was drafted into the army and sent to Vietnam, the couple suffered the only shaky period in their marriage. It was as if each one were infuriated with the other for not being able to protect their son from the possibility of harm. Mr. N's first heart attack drew them close together for a time, but when the news of their son's death reached them, they lapsed into a shell-like silence with each other, as if each one had given up on the other.

When her husband began to sail again, the patient felt as if she were somehow doomed to repeat her mother's life and her husband's destiny was bound to be intertwined with that of her father. One night she tried to break through the veil of silence that had shrouded the two of them since their son's death, but her words seemed like empty patter to her, despite the poignancy of the ideas she was voicing.

Early the next morning, Mrs. N's husband was hospitalized with the second heart attack, which was to claim his life, and she felt an immense burden of guilt for having ever brought up their silence. She clung to him with a ferocious tenacity in the hospital, hardly ever leaving his bedside, as if her bodily presence could force him to cleave to life and to her. "And then I went for a lousy cup of coffee, and he died. The son of a bitch. Why couldn't he have waited for me to get back? Why couldn't he have held on for ten damn minutes longer? Didn't he know that I loved him?"

Her tears in the session in which she described this to me mirrored the tears she had shed at his funeral and at the seemingly endless funerals that had preceded his. It required no special brilliance to connect the time of her husband's death with the onset of her alcoholism. Mrs. N readily acknowledged this fact, but the linkage once made, seemed to offer no especial remedy.

Although I was not privy to many of the details of Mrs. N's life during the consultative sessions, the sense of often repeated loss occurred again and again during the evaluation period. It appeared that whenever she found someone to be close to, they were "taken away" from her. Even those who were not especially close to her (such as her older brother and her mother), were also "taken away" from her. What made things worse, from her point of view, was that she was never there at their deaths. She was never even "given a chance" to verbalize any of the impassioned oratory she could have invented to make up for the earlier empty moments between them. Life kept dealing her "poker hands that were only fit to bluff with, and then called my bluff before I even got a chance to try to psych my opponent out. It sure as hell hasn't been fair." I had to agree with that appraisal of her life; it did not sound to me as if she had received a very fair deal either, although my agreement was made silently to myself.

Throughout the evaluation phase—some four or five sessions over a period of two and one-half weeks—I found no evidence of any of the important vegetative signs of depression. The tricyclic antidepressant medication her internist had prescribed for her was a more than adequate trial of the drug. My options then appeared to be to give her a trial on another antidepressant medication or to suggest to her that she might enter into analysis or analytic psychotherapy with me.

In our second meeting, in response to my question about any recent dreams she might have had, Mrs. N mentioned that she had been having some sad and disturbing dreams recently, only she could not really recall their content. She thought that, in one fragment she could recall, she had stretched out her arms to someone or something she could not quite reach. She was unable, however, to recall just whom or what it was that she was stretching toward.

The dream made her feel sad. "That's the story of my life," she observed. "The only people who were ever there for me were F (her husband) and R (her son) and they had to go and die, to put themselves out of my reach forever. And most of the other characters who made up the dramatis personae of my life were never really in my grasp at all." When she made these comments, she cried. Her tears, however, were followed by a good deal of the material previously described about her relationships with her father and her husband.

In the fourth session, which took place in the middle of February, she reported a fresh dream to me. "I think I was on a ship, a large yacht of the sort they use in the America Cup races. Only it was all draped in black, or at least everyone on board seemed to be dressed in black, as if they were in mourning for someone who'd died, someone important. I felt everyone's eyes upon me, as if I were supposed to be doing or saying something. Then I looked down at my clothes and they weren't all black, as the other people's were. It was as if they were made up of black and white stripes, like a kind of convict's garb. I felt shaky for a moment in the dream, as if I'd done something very wrong. Then I saw some of the people smiling kindly at me, and I felt steadier again. I think I grabbed onto the mast, too, to sort of prop myself up. I suppose it was a kind of crutch, but it felt so good to have something to hang onto."

In her associations to the dream, Mrs. N immediately related the important personage who had died to her father. "I guess I dreamt about him because we've been talking so much about all of the people who have died in my life. And it's Lincoln's birthday, too, isn't it? I think Whitman's poem *O Captain! My Captain!* was written for Lincoln's death, wasn't it? I remember having to stand up and recite that before the whole class in boarding school. There are some lines in there. . . ." Her voice trailed off for a moment and I strained forward to hear what she was saying. "It goes something like this, I think. . . ." And in a halting voice, almost totally drained of affect, she tossed off the better part of the dozen lines:

> Here Captain! dear father!
> The arm beneath your head!
> It is some dream that on the deck,
> You've fallen cold and dead.
> My Captain does not answer, his lips
> are pale and still,
> My father does not feel my arm, he
> has no pulse nor will,
> The ship is anchor'd safe and sound,
> its voyage closed and done,
> From fearful trip the victor ship
> comes in with object won;
> Exult O shores, and ring O bells!
> But I with mournful tread,
> Walk the deck my Captain lies,
> Fallen cold and dead.

We were both silent for a moment, pondering the meaning of the lines just rendered, and then she went on. "You know it's funny, I don't feel as saddened by all that as I suppose I should feel." I asked her what she meant by "should feel." "It seems obvious," she answered softly, "it's supposed to be a dream of mourning for the dead. I should be crying, only I don't feel like it right now. Maybe I've cried enough already. I'm probably just blocking off the feeling. I'm sure it'll come back later. But right now, it's as if I have a crutch to hang onto. I suppose that's you. You're the mast to anchor me in stormy seas. Strange thing was, it sounds funny to say it, in the dream I felt as if I were putting my hand around a tennis racket."

Little more emerged spontaneously to the dream and it was nearing the end of the session. "Any thoughts about being dressed in convict's clothing?" I asked.

"I wondered about that myself," she answered. "I suppose it has to do with feeling guilty and then everyone grants me a kind of absolution. I guess all of those sweetly smiling people must also represent you in some sort of way. I hope you don't mind being my crutch and my masthead right now. I need one badly." She was silent once more and then she added, just before the session ended: "You know, there was another poem I liked a lot in boarding school. It was William Ernest Henley's *Invictus*. The word convict is almost a play on it, on *Invictus*, someone who's invincible. I think it ends with the idea of being the captain of my fate and the master of my soul. That's what I'd like to end up with in here, being the captain of my own fate for a change, a little more invincible than I've been in the past, without conning myself into just thinking that I am."

I was deeply impressed with a number of features of the patient's response to the dream; even, I should say, to the presentation of the dream itself. I felt that important unconscious material was pushing itself forward in an ever-deepening fashion, as a result of the sessions we had already had. Moreover, by offering the dream to me and by the manner in which she had associated to it, Mrs. N was showing me that she possessed the capacity to participate actively in the treatment, regardless of the dependency (the crutch-like needs) being expressed.

Mrs. N's capacity to be an active participant in the treatment reminded me of Mr. T's. His ability to work with dreams and with the transference were also demonstrated early in the evaluative phase of the analysis. She indeed would like to be the captain of her own fate in reality. In addition, many of the important themes (tennis, father, probable phallic strivings, etc.) were readily available, as was the ability to recognize and not to shy away from working with the transference (seeing me as the smiling people and the ship's mast to anchor her). I saw these as very positive facets of Mrs. N's character structure.

The patient's obvious capacity for forming and for maintaining important object ties was another factor that led me to suggest to her that she undergo analysis. I made this recommendation, despite certain reservations about the depth of her depression (and the implicit wish for death and reunion with lost loved ones) and concerns about the physiological and psychological depth of her dependency on alcohol. Her wish to control her fate, her continuing potential for pleasure (as when she won a tennis match), and her ability to empathize with the need to spare her remaining brother any evidence of her drinking made me see her as a woman with considerable assets, despite the obvious liabilities she had exhibited.

Mrs. N's opening remark on the couch was an interesting one. "I guess it's my serve now," she said. "Let's see how many aces I can score in analysis." The implicit analogy made between the analysis and a tennis match also revealed her underlying competitiveness even more clearly than before. In response to this comment, I thought that besides wishing to grasp my tennis racket–crutch, Mrs. N might also want to wrest it away from me. In other words, I became aware of her castrative feelings toward men.

The patient returned to the theme of being one of the "least successful" people present at a party she had attended that night before. Again, the ideas of not being "with someone" and not "feeling lovable" were expressed in conjunction with a depreciation of herself. The person she most admired at the gathering was a rather tall, slender woman of a comparable age, who was present with her husband. Not only did she have an attractive husband, but she also had a career of her own in publishing. In addition, she had none of the excess weight about her middle that plagued the patient, and she was known at the country club as being an exceptional tennis player for her age, someone who could beat younger opponents with ease.

I noted to myself Mrs. N's feelings about my age (I was about 12 years younger). I then inquired about the other woman's being taller and slimmer than the patient was and was given to understand that these were generally desired qualities in our society. "But I guess that they do have an extra added attraction for me. If I looked like that, it'd make it a lot easier to feel that I was really different than my mother, or at least that I won't end up the same way that she did; fat, blotto, and dead."

From the patient's response, I came to see that the competitive motif she expressed in her opening remark was only one aspect of the total Gestalt of interlocking transference wishes she was expressing to me. Whether I was to give her a phallus or not (mine or someone else's), I was also to see to it that she would not turn out to be like her "blotto" mother, who essentially died alone and unloved. Needless to say, underneath the rejection of the mother lay the fear of, and wish for, a union with her in the transference, a fate seen as being tantamount to death, as well as to castration. Hence her desire to be the castrator, and not the one to be castrated.

"I just went home after the party and got drunk," Mrs. N continued. "Maybe I should just shut my mouth now and go to sleep on your couch. At least that way, I could get rid of my hangover." She was silent and when I inquired about her thoughts, she replied that all she could think about was how lousy she felt. Then she offered: "It seemed a little strange coming in here today. I really didn't know just what to expect." When I asked her whether or not her feelings about beginning the analysis might have had anything to do with her drinking too much the night before, her body instinctively flinched, as if she had been struck. "Ouch," she said, "I have the feeling that I could really get hurt in here. I'm not sure whether I like that very much. It's pretty scary."

Over the next few days and weeks, Mrs. N's sessions were crowded with references to her life. She talked about her attempts at socializing with friends and about her feelings of inadequacy in social situations, particularly when she compared herself with women who were married and/or those who had successful careers. Although there were occasional references to her mother's alcoholism, little material about her family or other aspects of her past emerged. In addition, the earlier allusions to the transference had all but disappeared. Then in one Friday session, just before a weekend break, I commented on the fact that most of her conversations in recent weeks had seemed to center upon present-day occurrences. She appeared irritated with me when she replied: "But you asked me to talk about whatever comes to my mind! And this is what's on my mind!"

Following this outburst, she was silent. Then she became briefly tearful. "Forgive me, doctor," she said, in a softer tone. "I'm just tired. I feel like hell today. I woke up this morning and I can't remember a damn thing about what happened last night. Please don't let me lose myself again. Don't let me go the route that she did. I couldn't stand myself if that were to happen to me. To forget a whole evening . . . it's a kind of craziness. . . . The thought of my being a goddam drunk is almost more than I can bear. Help me, doctor! Please God, help me!"

Mrs. N cried for several minutes and then attempted to dry her tears on the napkin on the bolster pillow on the couch. "I'll throw it out after the session," she commented. "It isn't right to make you handle this sopping mess. It's all smeared with tears and mascara now. It looks pretty horrible."

I suggested to her that she was obviously referring to more than just the napkin, that she must be feeling that way about herself at that moment. She nodded her head and began to cry again. When her sobbing ceased, I inquired about the wishes she had expressed that I prevent her from losing herself and that I not allow her to "go the route" her mother had gone. My question clearly led her away from the intensity of her feelings in the transference. I believe that I did this then, as I was beginning to wonder whether or not I had made a mistake in putting this patient on the couch. She responded to my inquiry by presenting a combination of historical and transference material. When the transference clearly began to predominate, I recognized my earlier wish to dilute its intensity and I resisted the temptation to repeat this maneuver again.

"I know it's supposed to be up to me," she said, "but in the scenario which I've prepared, you're there to keep me safe. You're supposed to stop me from drinking, so I'll always know who I am and what I've done. It's unholy to behave that way. Or maybe it makes me feel as if I'm full of holes."

Despite the covering joke about feeling full of holes, probably connected with a perception of herself as castrated, I was surprised by her utterance of the word, unholy, and I asked her about it. "It is an odd word," she acknowledged. "It sounds like a carryover from my church-going days as a kid. Daddy was an Episcopalian and mama was a Southern Presbyterian. . . . Most of the time we'd go with daddy, because mama wasn't in any shape to go with us. But once in a while we'd go with her and the minister in her church used to give these fire and brimstone type of sermons. He must have been a southerner like her. He was always talking about losing control and ending up in Hell out of sight of God forever. . . ." Her voice trailed off then, and became barely audible. As I strained to hear what she was saying, she murmured a bit more loudly: "God's supposed to be there for innocent little children, if they're good. Please be there for me, doctor. I promise to be good."

We were both quiet as we absorbed the content of what she had been speaking of. Then she went on: "I sounded just like her then. She used to talk to daddy like that, like a little child, when she'd get bombed on Sunday afternoon after church. She used to turn him into the preacher or into God, if he wasn't off sailing. It was just the way I tried to do it with you then. Oh sweet Jesus, I can't stand the thought of being like her. If I really thought that there were no way out, I'd kill myself."

The vehemence of her last utterance shocked me. I wondered again if I had been too cavalier in putting her on the couch. Then I felt angry, that she would be a disappointing patient, someone who would not measure up to my expectations. As I pondered these thoughts, which I quickly recognized as having a basis unrelated to the patient herself, I realized that my narcissistic defense was one I had used in response to certain disappointments with my own analyst. She, too, was a prototypical WASP, a woman Mrs. N reminded me of in a number of ways. The recognition helped me to abort the anger and the expectations I had been unconsciously imposing on the patient.

I also realized that I was being unconsciously placed by the patient in the position of being one of the important early objects in her life. I was thus expected to act out with her a sado-masochistic drama involving anger and rejection, with the latter being achieved either by verbal recriminations, which would presumably follow her drunken, infantile behavior, or by a silent withdrawal of my support. My impression was that I was being put in the position of the father interacting with the drunken mother on a Sunday afternoon. In this manner, although many different oedipal and pre-oedipal fantasies might be being enacted, my presumption was that she was most conspicuously acting out a fantasy of recovering her lost love objects (mother and father) by becoming like one (the mother) and turning me into another (the father).

I commented on how lonely she must have felt when she imagined herself to be forever out of the sight of God or of her parents. Then I wondered aloud about whether this feeling might have any especial intensity for her now, because of the impending weekend break in the analysis.

She began to cry again, and then said, "I will miss you a lot. I don't have anything planned at all for this weekend and my best friend's out of town for a couple of weeks visiting her daughter and grandchildren. I don't like being all by myself for so long a period of time, it's harder for me to avoid the drinking then."

"Maybe another way to put that," I noted, "would be to say that it's harder for you to stay 'good,' when you're all by yourself. And if you're not good, then maybe I won't be there for you." Part of me was tempted to add some such comment as "as your father wasn't there for your mother, when she was drunk," but I resisted the temptation. Although this again might have produced a flow of interesting genetic material, perhaps involving early anal accidents or conflicts over oedipal masturbatory fantasies (as exemplified in her current attitude toward the "messy" couch napkin), my prevailing belief was that this would not advance the analysis, since it would unnecessarily dilute the intensity of her transference feelings toward me.

"O,K., fine," she said, "so we've established that I need you. What am I supposed to do with my weekday crutch need when I'm not with you? Go to Lourdes and throw it away on weekends? I don't like the idea of being so dependent on you. You're not going to be there to take me home from the parties at night or to feed me black coffee in the morning to sober me up. What good are you really, you're either too much for me or not enough!"

In listening to her, I could see how she must have made her husband feel inadequate (as she so obviously felt herself to be) because he could not protect (or resurrect) their only son. How was he to guess that her criticisms of him stemmed (on one level) from her anger toward her father, both for his interactions with her directly and because of his inability to prevent the mother's alcoholism, and on another level toward her mother, for her inability to provide a consistent level of nurturing.

Throughout the course of the balance of the first year and one-half of the analysis, there were a number of alternating cycles in which the patient oscillated between periods of feeling closer to me in the transference with periods of acting distant and reserved. It gradually became apparent to both of us that she was re-enacting with me the alternating attitudes her mother had displayed toward her. The dual themes of my being both too much and not enough for her could be seen to be projections of her own feelings about herself vis-à-vis her mother, and about her mother herself. By being too much, she meant that she was a "bad, angry" child, who drove her mother to drink. By being "not enough," she referred to her inability to prevent her mother's alcoholism.

That the protestations directed against herself (as expressed toward me in the transference) could also be seen to be complaints against her inadequate parental objects also was quite apparent to us during this phase of the analysis. As this was clarified, the patient began to feel increasingly dependent on me and on the treatment. Unfortunately, however, Mrs. N's alcohol intake seemed to be little modified during this time and she still suffered from periodic blackouts, which upset her greatly and which led to intense outbursts of anger directed toward me because of my inability to prevent her drinking.

Shortly before the second summer vacation break, she brought in a dream that had awakened her the night after she had blacked out. "I was at a party with a group of people I didn't know. They all seemed to know each other and were all laughing and chattering away. No one talked to me, however, and I felt left out and I began to drink down one right after the other. Then you appeared, or at least somebody who looked like you appeared. I felt happy to see you and I touched you on the arm. Only you acted as if you didn't see me or hear me, or even feel my touch, as if I weren't even there somehow. I began to talk louder and to tug at your arm, only you still acted as though I weren't there. Then I began to scream and scream at you, to try to get your attention, and I woke up."

In her associations to the dream, Mrs. N quickly related her inability to "register" with me in any manner in the dream, with her current feelings of "impotence" with regard to getting me to respond to her needs. I reminded her of one of the "pod people" from a science fiction film, who snatched your body away, in the sense of assuming your exact likeness. Then they no longer registered any human emotions.

With respect to the action in the dream itself, it was as if I were the drunken one, not she. As if I were her mother, or even her father and older brother, all the people with whom she could never really "register" in her life. During the session in which she related these thoughts and feelings to me, she alternated between crying pitifully and giving vent to feelings of great anger to me. "I don't even touch you enough to make you want to stay here with me during August," she said, "even when you know how desperately I need you. You were supposed to make me invincible, but all you've done is to make me dependent on you and even weaker than I was before. I hate you for that! I hope you never come back!"

Mrs. N maintained her sense of anger and distrust of me in the remaining sessions before the summer break. When I returned in the fall, she had deep circles under her eyes, as if she had barely slept during the time that I had been away. "I've had a really rough time while you were away," she said, as if to confirm my worst impressions about her appearance. "I drank and drank, as if there were no tomorrow. And if I keep on like this, there won't be. The only thing that kept me focused in the slightest, was the notion of my coming in here today. I thought, if I can only make it till then, you'd make it well for me. Please make it well, doctor, I'm turning into an old lady before my eyes. I'm 56 now and I look like 80. What happens when I reach 60, if I ever get to live that long?"

To put it simply, this moment represented the nadir of the analysis. I seriously considered hospitalizing Mrs. N because of the severity of her drinking and the extent of her debilitation. I decided to tell her of my concerns for her well-being and I raised the question of putting her into the hospital.

"Whatever you think is best." Her voice had a beaten tone to it, as if she had surrendered to the inevitable (death) and were simply going through the motions of being alive. I felt touched by her despair and consciously wished to rescue her. I could also relate this wish to ones I had had in the past toward my former analyst and my own mother.

As a result of the warm feelings generated in me by the wish to rescue her, but with a considerable degree of trepidation, I informed the patient that, despite my concerns for her health and well-being, I still felt that it would be best for us to continue with the analysis. She seemed unaffected by my comments. Over the next few days, however, she began to look better.

"I hope you meant what you said the other day," she commented. "I don't want you to give up on me. That's what my father did with my mother and brother. He just gave up on them. And they died. I'm too scared to die now. Not while there's still nothing worth really living for. I don't want to die until I have something and am something. Only I need your help to keep me from slipping further into the abyss. You're the only handhold I've found in years. Don't let go of me now. Please don't let go of me."

When she reported these thoughts, my lack of responsivity to her touching me in the dream before the vacation break (her only handhold) seemed even more poignant. I commented on this and she agreed: "I tried to tell you that before you left. I didn't want you to go away last month. I knew it was going to be a bummer."

Over the next few months, Mrs. N began to act coquettish in our sessions. "I don't look so old anymore, do I?" She would ask. "I noticed some younger men casting lascivious glances at me in a restaurant the other day. What do you think of your old tennis partner now, doctor? I know, it's against the rules to answer. I only wish I had eyes in the back of my head to see the expression on your face. That'd be all the answer that I'd need."

In conjunction with these remarks, the patient began to rapidly shed the excess poundage that had plagued her for the past few years. "I haven't had a drink for three weeks now," she announced in the session before the Christmas break. "I've been a real good girl, haven't I? Don't you think that I deserve some kind of reward for that?"

When I asked her what her ideas were about the kind of reward she thought she deserved, she coyly answered that I ought to wrap myself up in tissue paper and give myself to her for Christmas. The playful request was repeated several times during the course of the session. She recalled her excitement as a child at Christmas, when she would eagerly anticipate the gifts her father would give her. Her tone of voice underscored the word father, as if to say that she knew that her mother had been too inebriated to select the gifts most of the time.

"When I was really young," she continued, "Christmas was one of the best times of the year for us. It was the only time of year when daddy really did anything special for us. The only time of year I ever really felt that he cared about me. I remember when he gave me my first tennis racket. I must have been no more than six or seven. I felt so proud to have one like he did, and my brothers did. I must've walked around beaming all day long, until my mother got drunk and almost knocked the Christmas tree over and fell and broke her wrist. That kind of deflated the rest of the day for me. She had a way of doing things like that, deflating days for me."

Mrs. N seemed pensive for a few moments, and I finally inquired about her thoughts. "I was just wondering why he stopped being close to me," she answered. "I must've been thirteen or fourteen, right before I went off to boarding school. He just sort of stopped the whole holiday routine. I felt bad about it, as if I'd done something and was being punished for it." Again she fell silent. Then, "I think it was about the time that my breasts began to develop and I got my period that he turned off. I've never thought of this before, but maybe he couldn't deal with the idea of my becoming a woman." As I started to ask her a question, she interrupted and said, "I know, you're going to ask me if maybe I was the one who had the sexual feelings toward him. That's such a strange thought. I can't even conceive of its being true."

I commented to her that perhaps it was not so strange a thought, inasmuch as she had put me in the place of her gift-giving father in her expressed wishes that I would wrap myself up in tissue paper and give myself to her for Christmas. My verbal underscoring of the word *give* italicized the sexual innuendo in her remark. In addition, I recalled for her several of the earlier sexual comments she had made to me.

"It's almost as if you're telling me that I shouldn't want you sexually," she said, "as if I really have done something bad and you're going to punish me by going away for Christmas." When I asked her about what she had just said, she became angry. "I know that you told me before that you are going away. I know that it has nothing to do with this, but it doesn't matter. The only thing that counts is that there's not a goddam thing that I can do to get you to spend the holidays with me or to get you to give me any piece of yourself that really counts, to hold onto while you're away. You really are an ungiving son of a bitch, just like my father was. He gave me a racket and then he never came to see me play. Maybe he couldn't stand seeing my tits shaking when I chased his balls. Jesus Christ, what am I saying? I sound like a textbook case of penis envy. Why the hell should I be giving you the Christmas present before you go? I'm the one who needs it."

It was only after my return from the holiday break that we were able to pursue the many themes that had arisen the session just before I left. I knew that I was "being punished," because the dark circles had returned beneath her eyes, telltale indicators that she had started drinking again.

"You're right," she said, attempting to read the expression on my face even before she lay down on the couch. "I drank a cup o' kindness then, to auld lang syne." We were both silent, and then she went on: "You try spending New Year's Eve by yourself, or Christmas day. It's not a terrific feeling." Suddenly the anger and the mockery drained from her voice. "God I missed you! I think I got drunk because I hated myself so bad for wanting you sexually. I just wanted to blot the whole feeling out, to drown it in alcohol."

The next day, she pursued the theme again: "I don't know, it was so many different things. I felt like you'd taken the essential me with you when you went away, whatever that means. Plus whatever warm, sexual, female part I have left in my being. And I guess you did chop off my balls, too, just the way that he used to do when he wouldn't come to see me play tennis. You ought to play football, doctor, you're really a triple threat man."

In the months that followed, we unraveled many of the tangled threads from these themes and we learned a great deal about her feelings of conflict over having been born a girl and of her envy of her brothers. Despite her recognizing that her father had not been able to give any more emotionally to her brothers than to her, Mrs. N still clung to the fantasy that he would have found her more lovable if she had been a boy. She revealed that she had had considerable difficulty achieving orgasms during intercourse with her husband and with her prior lovers and had only been able to do so with the aid of a fantasy of being humiliated sexually at the hands of men who were obvious surrogates for the father. She further confessed that she had been masturbating to orgasm for some time now, while utilizing similar fantasies involving me.

As we worked through some of this difficult material, there were brief episodes of "breaking the fast," as Mrs. N put it, where she would drink heavily. But as the third summer vacation break drew closer, she had not been drinking for approximately six weeks.

"I'm worried," she said, "I don't know if I can stay off while you're away. Last summer stands out like such a horror show in my memory. I don't want to repeat the same disaster again this time."

She spoke of the wish to make me feel guilty about hurting her, to make me feel responsible for her drinking, as she had felt herself to be responsible for her mother's. "O.K.," she announced before I left, "I'll let you go now and I won't hurt myself. But hurry back before I change my mind."

When I returned in the fall, she showed none of the physical signs of the heavy drinking of the prior summer. I felt as if we were beginning to see progress. In a sense, this perception was correct. Even though the patient had once more contrived to dilute the intensity of the painful transference feelings she was experiencing, this time it was without the aid of alcohol.

What Mrs. N had managed to do was to resurrect the tenuous relationship with her remaining brother. By examining their interaction, we were able to see that she was attempting to undo the narcissistic mortifications suffered at the hands of the rejecting analyst by displacing her feelings of warmth (and of sexual desire) onto him. She realized that she probably had done the same thing with him as a teenager, when the father had rejected her, only to come a cropper with her brother, also, when he had married. He had always been spared the anger she had felt for the father, however, because of the unfortunate course of his married life and because of the warmth he had offered her in her adolescent time of need.

The upsurge of closeness to the brother remained, even though she recognized it as reflecting her need to undo the feeling of trauma suffered at my hands in the transference. They met some rather important nurturing and quasi-sexual and social needs for each other at that time, and both of them appeared reluctant to question this type of gratification and to risk further "wounds" by venturing forth into any other relationships.

As the year passed, little analytic work was accomplished and I began to wonder if the treatment would stalemate. In the springtime, however, early in the fourth year of the treatment, Mrs. N came in one day and announced: "I saw D [her brother] last night and he told me that he's been seeing a woman I know, for the last few weeks. He said that he liked her a lot. I felt incredibly jealous when he told me about her. She was a classmate of mine in boarding school and she's still a strikingly pretty woman. She and her husband split up a few years ago and I've seen her at the club quite a bit since then. She's the kind of woman who always manages to attract more than her share of men without any trouble, as if she sends out some kind of signal to them and they respond to it." She was pensive for a moment and then added, "I've often wondered what sort of woman your wife is, whether she's pretty or sexy. I guess I mean is she prettier and sexier than I am. God, that was hard to say!"

With this beginning revelation of her competitive desire to replace my wife, Mrs. N's sexual fantasies came more clearly into focus in the next year of analysis. She was reluctant to reveal these fantasies to me, inasmuch as they made her feel "defective" and "inadequate" vis-à-vis her presumed picture of my wife. In these ongoing masturbatory epics, she was most often depicted as being forced to strip naked before a group of men in a large room or amphitheatre. Then she would be made to lie down upon a cold examining table and would have to put her legs up in a pair of gynecological stirrups, while a doctor dressed in a white coat exposed her vagina and clitoris to the gaze of these men, who would then proceed to have intercourse with her.

In her associations to these fantasies, I was clearly seen as the doctor–father who was humiliating her. She also spoke of her perception of her genitals as "ugly" and "damaged" and only half-mockingly verbalized her desire to have a "tennis racket and tennis balls" between her legs, as brother D and I did, so that she could find someone attractive to make love to.

When I questioned her about the homosexual desires implicit in her statement, she spoke of feeling "anxious" and "exposed," which she related once more to the content of her fantasies. "In some of them," she observed, "there's a woman standing there in the midst of the men. She's tall and slim, like all the women I've ever admired. I suppose," she added, semi-pandering to me," she's the woman with the penis whom I've always longed to be. I suppose that could be true, only I think it's got to be more than just that."

Her associations dried up then, and only some weeks later, when the subject arose again, were we able to pursue it further. "My mother was a sloppy drunk," she announced one day. "She'd toss and turn a lot in her bed and then she'd lie there with her nightgown gathered up around her head. It used to bother me, seeing her naked that way. I felt embarrassed for her, being open like me and to my brothers. I hated her indifference to the way that she looked and acted. But at the same time, I remember wanting to cover her over with my own body, to protect her from being looked at by the wrong eyes."

"The wrong eyes?" I asked.

"From them," she responded. "From me, too, I guess. Oh God, I don't even want to think about what you're getting at, of my wanting her that way. It's repulsive to want to sleep with your own mother. I know that it was more than just something sexual that I wanted with her. I think it was a way of healing her wounds, our wounds, of making her whole again, making both of us whole. I know, I know . . . I wanted to be her penis . . . so we'd both be perfect and there'd be no need for her to stay drunk all day and to try to fill up the bottomless hole in her mind. And then maybe my father would've stayed home and not been out in the city till all hours, and my older brother would've still been alive and God knows what else would've happened." Mrs. N was quiet for a few moments; then she continued: "I was almost trying to put all that stuff down as I said it, just now, but you know, I think there's really a lot of truth in all of it."

I told her that I, too, thought that there was a great deal of truth in it. I reminded her of how the idea of being made whole, by having me serve as her penis, had come up frequently before times of separation in the analysis, and of how the loss of her son and of her husband had intensified her feelings of emptiness and incompleteness and had led to her drinking, in an identification with her lost mother and brother. As we began to work more thoroughly through many of these themes in the fifth year of the analysis, the patient was finally able to mourn her lost loved objects adequately and to ease the heavy burden of guilt she had been carrying around for many years. As she accomplished this, her drinking ceased to be an issue in the analysis.

Early in the sixth year of the treatment, Mrs. N announced that she had been offered a job doing public relations work for a firm in her local area. "It'll be just part time to start," she said, "but it's a great opportunity and if I'm successful and the business takes off as they think it will, they told me they'd offer me a full time job in the fall."

We both recognized that this job would make it virtually impossible for her to attend her sessions as frequently. Initially, it meant cutting our sessions from four a week to three. But in the fall, she thought, we would probably have to cut back even further or even perhaps stop altogether. We pursued quite thoroughly the question of whether or not the idea of taking a job represented another attempt to dilute the intensity of the transference feelings. Although there was a certain degree of truth in this idea, the motivations in opting for this excellent job opportunity seemed to be closely bound to reality, such as her age (she was almost 60) and the quality of the job vis-à-vis her lack of real business experience. We decided to try to accomplish as much work as possible by the summer vacation break and in the fall we would determine whether we should continue with the treatment.

Mrs. N felt happy with the tentative termination decision. She spoke of her sadness at leaving me and the analysis and was able to recognize her identification with the father, both in the choice of business she was entering and in the idea of leaving someone behind to wait for her (analyst–mother). She was glad that I was "always going to be there," because I was younger than she was and would likely die after she did. With this latter thought (her real consideration of her age and of her concerns about dying), we ushered in the final phase of the analysis. Here, the dual themes of being able to separate from a love object while still retaining one's capacity to remain alive, on one hand, and to feel complete and separate, on the other, were of paramount importance. In her masturbatory practices, and in her occasional relationships with men, her need for her fantasies of being humiliated to attain orgasm was much attenuated. In general, the patient felt a great deal better about herself, particularly as her job turned out to be a glowing success.

She then began to work full time and decided to terminate the analysis, though she did pay me a series of visits before the holidays that year. "I thought of wrapping myself up in tissue paper," she said jokingly, "I'm a pretty good advertisement for the efficacy of analysis. If I ever found my own firm, I think I'll call it Invictus. I may not really be totally invincible against the threats of losing someone I care about or of dying, but I've come a long way in that direction. If I'm not totally the captain of my fate, I've certainly reached the rank of first lieutenant."

At this juncture, let me once more comment on some of the important points illustrated by this particular case. For one thing, it is of interest to note that the general course of the analysis here seemed to differ very little from that of a younger person. That the patient was in her middle 50's when treatment began seemingly had little effect on the nature of the material produced. I see this as a further piece of evidence for a point commented on in the case of Mr. T, that is, the age of the patient is not of paramount significance, but rather the nature of the psychopathology and the facets of the character structure are.

A second facet of the case was the degree of success obtained in dealing with the patient's severe drinking problem. Alcoholism is a syndrome that, in my own experience, is notoriously unresponsive to psychoanalytic intervention, even in patients considerably younger than Mrs. N. Why she should have responded so well is not an easy question for me to answer.

In Mrs. N's case, the very fact of her being older and more concerned with the issues of aging and death was of great significance with regard to her ultimately giving up drinking. What made this especially poignant for her was that, regardless of her unconscious wish to rejoin her mother (the lost love object) through death, her fears of the destructive nature of these wishes prevailed and intensified her motivation for treatment. That she was approaching the age at which her mother had died was an important factor in both getting her into treatment initially and in keeping her in it through the early demoralizing years, but it was hardly the only factor. What I wish to underscore here is that the nature of the relationship established in my patient's mind between her own age, and the age at which her mother died, raised her anxiety at a number of different fantasy levels. It represented both an oedipal triumph (if she lived past the age of her mother's death) and also the realization of a preoedipal wish for fusion and reunion (if she died at the same age). These fantasies, which were important to Mr. T also, were especially important for Mrs. N because they represented a potentially concrete realization of these important unconscious wishes.

This realization seems to function in a patient such as this as a day residue might in the formation of a dream. It appears to bring important unconscious fantasies to the surface. These then act as a mini-traumatic neurosis, which keeps pressuring for relief and resolution through symptom formation or overt actions. Obviously, such an explanation is, at best, incomplete.

Finally, let me note that the case of Mrs. N, like that of Mr. T, demonstrates the ability of the older patient to deal with difficult psychodynamic, genetic, and transference material with the ease of a younger patient. Although the major symptomatic resistance was a frightening one (her alcoholism), which almost caused me to abort the analysis, we were able to work it through and to achieve a salutory result.

4
THERAPY OF A VIRGINAL WOMAN: Ms. B

When I first saw Ms. B, she was a 55-year-old woman with rather closely cropped, brownish-blonde hair, lightly streaked with flecks of gray, and an almost chalkily pale skin drawn tautly across her high cheekbones; the areas beneath her clear blue eyes and across her forehead were marked by occasional age lines. Objectively, her face and body were younger than her stated age, but the sense of expectancy she communicated lent a feeling of urgency to her persona—a feeling that smacked of disquiet and dissatisfaction. Although she was not overtly sexual in her dress and conversation, the directness of her gaze and the intensity of her manner led me to believe that she had a considerable degree of warmth, perhaps even of passion. It came as no great shock, however, when she informed me that she was still, technically, a virgin.

"I had a hysterectomy about six months ago," she said, "for bleeding fibroids. I told my gynecologist that as long as he was cleaning me out down below, he might as well open me up, too, since I was still a virgin. It took me a while to get over the surgery, but now that I feel better, the reason I'm here is to ask you to help me get opened up and cleaned out up above, as well."

I smiled to myself when she talked. I had not quite expected this type of speech in her presenting complaints. In addition, what she said seemed to attest to a degree of pluckiness, that positively disposed me toward her. Her comments also had a sound of solidity behind them, a solidity of purpose that bespoke the depth of her motivation for treatment. She seemed like someone who genuinely wanted to change herself because she was not the kind of person she wished to be.

Historically, a cloud had hung over Ms. B's life since birth. Less than 72 hours after her birth, her 28-year-old mother had died of pulmonary emboli from a thrombophlebitic leg, caused by a broken leg in the final month of her pregnancy. Family legend had it that Ms. B had continued to nurse at her mother's breast even after her mother had died, despite the fact that the mother had apparently cried out (a fact attested to by a passing nurse in the hospital corridor) and let go of the infant as her arms flailed out in death. Whether apocryphal or not, the story was intrinsically woven into the patient's myth of herself, in a manner that seemed to her a glaring testimony of her own innate "greediness."

The patient had been the only child of the union between her parents. Although her mother had been described to her as a bright, attractive woman, apparently the marriage had not been a happy one. Legend once more had it that the patient's conception had been planned to shore up the marriage. With the mother's death, the father, who had been involved in a series of illicit liaisons before the patient's birth, sullenly gave up his affairs. Unfortunately, however, he seemed to hold his infant daughter responsible for the termination of these liaisons, which had afforded him the only real pleasure he had apparently known with women. Thus, the patient was doubly stigmatized from birth. On the one hand, she held herself responsible for her mother's death (reasoning that the mother would never have slipped and broken her leg if she had not been pregnant), and on the other, she saw herself as the "cause" of her father's unhappiness. Although she never consciously verbalized these thoughts, she seemed to have lived her life as if they were the motive force of her existence.

After his wife's death, Ms. B's father buried himself in his work and withdrew from social contacts for a number of years. He channeled his energy, creativity, and love into designing and erecting the houses he built as an architect and contractor in the town in which he and his daughter lived. The patient was raised by her maternal grandmother, who had been living with the young couple at the time of the patient's mother's death. The grandmother, a widow in her late 50's, was hardly a font of warmth and love. The death of her daughter (an only child), had followed, by 18 months, the death of her husband. Although she was grudgingly grateful to her son-in-law for providing her with a home, she disapproved of his morality and character. Her presence in the home, moreover, constantly reminded Ms. B's father of his earlier infidelities. It is unlikely that the father would have long tolerated his mother-in-law's silent censure, had it not been useful to have her care for his infant child. Thus, the household could hardly be characterized as a happy, nurturing one.

Shortly after Ms. B's fourth birthday, the grandmother was discovered to be suffering from cancer and underwent the first of a series of operations so that she was away from the household for weeks and often months at a time. A number of young farm girls were tried out in the position of housekeeper and surrogate mother for the child, but the patient's father found them all inadequate and one succeeded another.

On the day of the patient's fifth birthday, her grandmother returned from the hospital for what was to be her last stay at home. Ms. B was thrilled to see her grandmother and the feelings seemed to be mutual. The little girl cuddled up next to the older woman in bed and fell asleep. When the father walked in, his pent-up rage at the child exploded and he yanked the little girl rudely out of the bed and screamed out at her that she would soon be the death of her grandmother as well, because of her greedy selfishness. The child, horrified at the threat of the prospective loss, slunk from the room in guilty terror. When the grandmother died, some six months later, her death was added to the lengthening list of crimes for which the little girl held herself responsible.

Without his mother-in-law's presence, the patient's father once more reverted to philandering. On two or three occasions, Ms. B found him in bed with one of the farm-girl housekeepers when she went to see if her father was up and ready to take her to church on Sunday. She felt confused by these discoveries and worried that her father might be held responsible for the death of one of the girls, since it was obvious to her that being in bed with someone was tantamount to wanting to kill them.

The coup de grace was delivered to the patient shortly after she began to go to school, early in her seventh year. Her father announced that he was remarrying. He had chosen a person considerably younger than himself (a woman in her early twenties) who had little interest in mothering another woman's child and who wanted children of her own, to cement her marriage to this prominent architect and builder. In addition, the stepmother reasoned, if her husband had a happy family life (not the previous morbid one) he might remain faithful to her. When the stepmother gave birth to first one girl (when the patient was 8) and then another (when Ms. B was 10), it became obvious to the patient that little nurturing was to come from anyone within her home.

When Ms. B was 11, her teacher that year turned out to have considerable talent as a ceramicist and glassmaker. Ms. B became an ardent admirer and imitator of her teacher's work, and would often visit her after school to watch her in her studio. The teacher's husband was a pleasant man, but the young girl seemed excessively shy in his presence and he recognized that the child's interest was in being close to his wife. He knew about the tragic circumstances surrounding her birth and about the succession of ill-suited housekeepers, and he felt sorry for her. He also knew how her stepmother neglected her.

For one of the very few times in her life, Ms. B felt genuinely liked by other people. In her fantasies, she openly substituted the admired teacher and her husband for her stepmother and father. In an elaborate and ongoing daydream, she became their real daughter. Her new mother was discovered by the critics and was lauded as a great artist, and her works were sought after by the museums in New York City. The three of them would ride the train into the city and visit the Metropolitan Museum and the patient would glow with pride as people admired her mother's works. On rare occasions, one of Ms. B's daydreams might include a sequence in which a museum or gallery might opt to include one of her own works in a novel mother–daughter exhibit. Even then, she deferred to the works of her "mother," but her own productions were reviewed favorably by the art critics. These sequences, in the ongoing surrogate family saga, generally followed an episode of especial praise for a work of the patient's by her teacher.

Occasionally, the patient would introduce a note of anxiety into the daydreams. Something would go wrong with a shipment of their creations, and the art would be misplaced. At such times, the surrogate father would intercede and everything would turn out well. He was the protector, the man who took care of things and of the women he loved. Whether in the happy or in the anxious form, the ongoing fantasies gave the patient a great deal of pleasure and she passed much of her time elaborating them. In the fantasies, at least, the world about her was populated with loving family members. The contrast with her actual family life thus became increasingly apparent.

When the school year ended, and the patient moved into another class, the relationship with the admired teacher seemed in jeopardy. At that time, however, reality became nearly congruent with the fantasies, when the teacher and her husband (who were unable to have children) invited the patient to spend the summer with them at an art colony upstate. Her father and stepmother willingly gave their permission, and the young acolyte went off with her surrogate parents for the summer.

It was an idyllic time, filled with long discussions of art and poetry and even longer walks through the mountains and by the lakes of the beautiful countryside. Ms. B prayed that the summer would never end and that the happy days and nights would go on forever. But the time for the return home came and was marked indelibly in the young pupil's mind by the advent of her menarche. She was fortunate in having her teacher there to explain it to her, but even with the woman's loving initiation into the rites of womanhood, Ms. B felt her daydreams rudely shattered. Now she, too, must marry, mate, give birth and die, as her real mother had. Life was cruel, she thought, to allow her to partake of the fruits of happiness and then to steal them away from her again so quickly.

The loving teacher and her husband attempted to maintain the close ties they had established with the patient. Despite her apprehensions that all that went before was to have gone for nought, she allowed herself to be drawn into the loving circle of their home and hearth on many occasions throughout the next two years. Under the tutelage of her mentor, she became an accomplished artist and drew the praise of a number of the adults in her hometown, with the notable exception of her father and stepmother, who, although they paid little attention to her, still seemed to be oppressed by her presence in their household. After she finished grade school, she was packed off to an exclusive girl's boarding school in another state, over her own objections and those of the former teacher and her husband.

At this school, Ms. B felt a social leper. She had always been ill at ease with her peers and the disparity in social expertise that separated her from most of her schoolmates only served to accentuate her unease. In addition, she sorely missed her surrogate parents and their demonstrative love and affection. She was lonely and isolated, and her art, which had previously helped her express her innermost feelings, seemed out of place in a school where one's social prestige paralleled one's prowess in field hockey. Night after night, Ms. B cried herself to sleep. The headmistress of the school spoke with her on a few occasions and even telephoned her father once or twice, but mostly she was left on her own to unhappiness. The patient became even more isolated when her classmates entered a round of debutante parties from which the patient was excluded because of her father's disinterest in such matters.

For a brief period, Ms. B attempted to fit in with the other girls. She tried field hockey, but was a poor player and was made fun of by the other students. The one or two students she struck up relationships with were yanked out of school by their families. Again, she turned back to her art and revived the fantasies about her idealized teacher-mother and the teacher's husband-father. She continued to see them whenever she could, but there was just too much time between visits home to counteract her loneliness at school.

Soon the time came for the patient to make up her mind as to a career. At the suggestion of her beloved teacher, Ms. B spoke with her father about the possibility of going to a state teacher's college to study to become an art teacher.

For the only time in her memory, Ms. B's father spoke with her at length about her proposed career plans. He showed more concern in this one conversation then he had shown in the previous 18 years of her life. She was surprised at the perceptiveness of his questions and the depth of his understanding of the genesis of her interest in art.

"I haven't been a good father," he said, after they had talked about her teacher's concern for her future. "I always blamed you for your mother's death and I'm sorry for that. I didn't mean to yell at you that time with your grandmother, and to call you greedy. I think I was really blaming you for my own shortcomings. It wasn't that I really loved your mother, either. I'm sure you've heard all that before. It's common enough knowledge around this town. But when she died, I was vilified in the eyes of the people we knew. Maybe in my own eyes as well. And somehow you came to stand for the concrete representation of my sins. . . ."

As her father spoke to her, Ms. B stared directly into his eyes, as if she were looking at him for the first time. She did not know how she had the courage to stare at him so intently, but she had.

"I don't really love your stepmother either, you know," her father continued. "She's a nice enough person, but she's a Lilliputian when it comes to carrying on a conversation. I think I always wanted someone I could talk to, someone I could share my dreams and my desires with. Your mother always made me feel guilty about them, as if I were some sort of pariah for having them. But it wasn't really her fault, her being that way. She just wanted an ordinary kind of man. And I'm not an ordinary kind of anything. I never allowed myself to turn to you to help meet my needs. I guess I cheated both of us by that omission. I'm sorry."

Ms. B felt at a loss for words when the conversation lapsed. It was one thing to talk with her art teacher or her teacher's husband, but quite another to talk with her father. And especially when he seemed to want something from her, something she felt ill prepared or unable to give. The words "I forgive you, daddy," flashed across her mind for an instant, but her courage failed her and she remained silent.

"I don't know why I'm burdening you with all of this now," her father said, "it must be because you're going away again. And maybe you won't be coming back, this time. I have a funny kind of presentiment that we're never really going to get a chance to talk again. I know that sounds melodramatic, but I just believe it'll turn out to be true. Maybe I just don't want you to hate me, even if you never do get to know me."

When her father had first begun to unburden himself, Ms. B had wondered if he would suggest that she not go off to school. But then she realized that he would not try to interfere. She felt uneasy when her father spoke of his feelings that they might not get the chance to talk so personally again. His feelings of guilt toward her had been a revelation, and she did not know quite what to make of his statements. Maybe over a period of time they could talk more to each other and resolve some of their misunderstandings. As the conversation ended, her father placed his hand over hers. It was the first time in her life, that the patient ever recalled his touching her with anything like affection. Her eyes misted over, but she quickly looked down, so that her father might not see this lapse of control and be offended.

At the state teacher's college, Ms. B found other women who shared her interests in art. She could talk to them about her own ideas and theories about various subjects and was pleased when no one laughed at her. She wrote to her former teacher and spoke of how much pleasure she would experience at the practice teaching placements with the local school children in the city where she was studying. She even wrote a few awkward letters to her father that first fall, and he answered her, but neither one of them could open up in this medium.

Just before Ms. B was to have gone home for the Christmas holidays, she was informed that her father and stepmother had been killed in an auto crash. Her father had apparently been drinking at a party at a friend's home and had lost control of his automobile on the way home. Her stepmother had been killed immediately and her father had died shortly after arriving at the local hospital (where her mother had died).

When the patient heard this, a sense of blankness enveloped her. In retrospect, she recalled that she felt as if the light had gone out of her life for a moment and then slowly returned, but with a lower wattage. At the funeral, she felt detached from herself, as if she were envisioning herself from afar, going through the motions. Only for a moment or two on that terrible day did the observing and participating aspects of her self-representation come together. When they did, she cried convulsively for a short time, but she soon regained her composure and the welcome sense of detachment from her feelings. Her state of depersonalization lasted, on and off, for the better part of 48 hours, when it went away and she became depressed. She felt a sense of overwhelming loss and cried inconsolably. She even felt sorry for her stepsisters, but they drew their source of comfort from their maternal grandparents, with whom they would be living.

After the reading of her father's will, which provided her with sufficient funds to pursue her studies and to ultimately live comfortably off the income from his investments, Ms. B visited her teacher and her husband. The loving couple tried to console the patient, but did not understand the nature of her feelings. She had never told them about the poignant conversation with her father or about the letter writing. They were surprised that she felt so bereft; he had been so mean to her, they reasoned, she really should not grieve him quite so deeply. Perhaps they were jealous of her attachment to her father. When the patient finally posed that question in her treatment with me, there was no way to answer it definitively.

Ms. B went back to college and continued her studies. She withdrew from her friends for a long while and did not feel quite as thrilled about her upcoming teaching placements. Ultimately, however, she began to feel enthusiastic about her ceramics and her glassblowing again. She tried to paint in oils, but eventually gave this up, since she felt that she could not express herself in this medium. Only during her treatment did we come to recognize this endeavor as an attempt to effect a greater degree of separation between herself and the surrogate mother–art teacher of her childhood.

For a brief period, Ms. B toyed with the idea of becoming an architect like her father, but the thought was never a serious one. When she finally turned to photography, she knew she had found her real metier. Even though she knew she would never excel at it, she loved it and pursued it with an intensity she would not have dreamed possible. Some of her photographs were printed in the college magazine, and a few in the local newspaper. She was thrilled by this and wished that she could show the papers to her father, only he was dead. Whenever she had such thoughts, she would cry. Why had their relationship been aborted, just as it was starting? Consciously, she could find no way to blame herself for his death, though unconsciously she once more linked his death with his fleeting closeness to her.

Although Ms. B's guilt feelings (and her perception of herself as a carrier of a deadly plague that infected everyone who came close to her) managed to keep her from forming any close attachments to anyone, they did not prevent her from pursuing her career. She graduated from college with her degree as a teacher and was determined to impart her own knowledge to others who also were interested in learning about photography and art. She invited her former teacher and her husband to her graduation, but they were unable to come because her mentor was too weak to make the trip. She had been diagnosed as suffering from carcinoma of the lung some months before, and by the time Ms. B saw her, she was obviously dying. The patient maintained a vigil at her teacher's bedside, alternating with the husband, who seemed more resigned to his wife's loss than the patient did. Only Ms. B, however, was at the bedside when her mentor died. She grasped the frail body in her arms and attempted to infuse some of her own life spirit into it, but to no avail. As fate would have it, when the nurse entered the room, Ms. B was found crying with her head pressed against her former teacher's breast, in an ironic reprise of the earlier scene with her real mother.

After the funeral, Ms. B spent some time with her former teacher's husband. She had always been fond of the man and had looked upon him as a father surrogate. He, too, was a teacher, but in a very different area. At the man's house, after the mourners left, they talked of many things, mostly of the times the three of them had spent together, as in the summer at the art colony. She felt a sense of warmth toward her companion and sensed that he felt it too. When he spoke about how lonely he was, she understood his mood. She had felt that way herself so many times in the past. But when he awkwardly embraced her and tried to kiss her, she felt confused at first, and then fearful and angry. It was not right, she thought, it seemed to violate the moment and her trust in him. The man, too, seemed confused and for a fleeting instant the patient wondered just what to do; she then left the house and never saw him again. It was as if the last ties with her past had been broken and she could now go her own way.

She packed her bags and took the train to New York City. When she arrived, she found rooms and obtained a job teaching at one of the city schools, where she felt at home almost immediately. Although the school somewhat resembled the boarding school she had gone to, it differed significantly from that place: the students were more like herself, caught up with a desire for learning and the pursuit of art, rather than being preoccupied with athletics. Many were lonely children and she saw them as kindred spirits. Class after class took a liking to her, and she became one of the more popular teachers in the school.

Though she never verbalized anything about the encounter with her former teacher's husband, it seemed clear to us later that this episode had driven her even further from the possibility of any contact with a man. The quasi-incestuous overtones of the encounter had upset her, as had the subliminal perception of her own desires. And somewhere in the back of her mind stood the specter of her perception of herself as being too deadly to allow anyone to make the mistake of getting close to her. Thus, the decision was slowly made to live alone and to devote her life to teaching.

Over the years, Ms. B did date a few men, but none of these relationships were of any consequence. Whenever any one of them made a sexual advance, she would rebuff him and stop dating him. As she described these abortive interactions with men during our initial sitting-up sessions, they seemed more to reflect her fear of the consequences of allowing anyone to get really close to her, than any real aversion to sexuality. In addition, her fear of becoming pregnant, and of consequently giving birth, was another important determinant of the apparent shallowness in her relationships with men.

"I know it sounds a little stupid," she said, "but I'm certain that I always felt that if I had a baby, I would die the way my mother had done with me. As if fate would demand that from me, as retribution for her death. I don't know why I was never able to shake that fear, but I couldn't. It was only when I finally had the hysterectomy that I felt safe. . . . That's when I decided to ask the doctor to open me up, so I'd be able to sleep with a man if I wanted to. I regret that I'll never be able to have a child, to see how good a mother I could have been, but the fear of fate was too great. Besides, it's too late now for regrets."

The concreteness of Ms. B's reasoning bothered me. It was as if she had been unable to separate the fantasy of retaliation for her mother's death, from the reality of it. I was bothered by this difficulty of hers because I had been seriously entertaining the possibility of analyzing her, despite her age and the difficulties in her object-relationships over the years. But I did not know just how traumatized she was from her early life events and the erratic nurturing she had received from the significant adults in her immediate family. Essentially, I did not know if she had a sufficiently strong observing ego to allow her to distinguish between transference and reality.

When I began to compare the pros and cons of analyzing Ms. B, I realized that they seemed quite "iffy." There were a number of factors against her being analyzable. Perhaps the prime difficulty would be the depth of her masochism and of the need to punish herself for her presumed transgressions against her mother, father, and grandmother. Although her father's poignant conversation with her before she went off to college had somewhat muted her conscious feelings of guilt, it had only really scratched the surface.

Along with the guilt and the need to punish herself was the question of the intensity of her rage toward others. Had this been the truly limiting factor in her relationships with men? Obviously, her perception of herself as a modern day Typhoid Mary was really a defense that blocked her recognition of herself as a destructively angry person. Would her rage surface in the transference and affect her ability to perceive me as separate and distinct from the destructive father of her early childhood? If it did, would she develop a psychotic transference that might be unanalyzable?

In another vein, although Ms. B denied any episodes of depersonalization other than the one that had occurred after the death of her father, I wondered if her memory was quite accurate. Might not this defensive distortion of specific functions of the ego prevent her perception and integration of intense affects in the transference? Needless to say, I had no ready answers to my questions or to my nagging concerns about the patient.

On the positive side of the issue of whether or not the patient was analyzable, a number of facts stood out. For one thing, there had been a number of positive nurturing figures in Ms. B's past. Her maternal grandmother, depressed as she was, apparently had loved the little girl. In addition, a number of the young farm-girl housekeepers also seemed to have been rather warm, loving figures. And certainly her surrogate mother–schoolteacher, as well as the teacher's husband, were the most important nurturers in the line of adult figures in Ms. B's life. We later came to see that a thinly disguised version of the teacher's husband entered the patient's occasional masturbatory fantasies. I did not know this at the time of the evaluation, but simply knew that she had masturbated to orgasm with fantasies of different men. Hence her sexual inhibition did not seem to be absolute.

In listening to the patient's description of her interactions with the teacher and her husband, and of their long conversations about art and poetry, I had the strong impression that Ms. B had formed a deep object tie with them. To my mind, this meant that her capacity for effecting such ties had not been destroyed. Furthermore, she had formed a number of significant relationships with women during her college years and had maintained them throughout her life. She had also formed close relationships with women throughout her teaching career, and relationships with both men and women who shared her artistic interests. In other words, even though her capacity for achieving close emotional ties were limited, such ties were not impossible.

In her work, the patient led a happy, successful life. She loved teaching and was accorded to be excellent at it by her peers and students. Indeed, a number of young pupils of hers seemed to have owed the inspiration for their own pursuit of artistic careers to her. Although she never received the rave notices from the critics she had longed for, she was a modest success in art circles. Most important of all, from my point of view, she took a great sense of pride and pleasure in her work and in that of her pupils. She positively seemed to glow as she spoke of her teaching and her art work and the legacy she imparted to her pupils. In listening to her, I felt that she had great untapped reservoirs of passion and pleasure that might also be directed toward relationships with people if the treatment were successful.

Finally, I noted a pluckiness (or courage) which had been manifested in her staring directly at her father (confronting him, so to speak, despite his previous rejections of her) when she was discussing her career plans and in her decision to go to New York City. It was also evident in her handling of her hysterectomy and in the way she spoke of wanting to be "opened up," both down below and up above, of really wanting "to change," which bespoke a strong motivation. The only area in which she was lacking was in her interactions with men. And this was one of the reasons she had come to see me. Specifically, she had asked her gynecologist to refer her to a male psychiatrist because she had wanted to confront directly a representative of the sex she had had the most trouble with in her life.

When I finally suggested the idea of analysis to her, and mentioned the utilization of the couch and the frequency of the visits, Ms. B became quiet and contemplative. "It sounds as if it's a very lonely kind of treatment," she finally noted. "I'm not sure that's what I really bargained for in here. I thought of our confronting things more directly, kind of looking at them, at each other." She hesitated for a few moments and then continued: "But maybe what you're saying to me is that if I relive the loneliness in here with you, I'll understand more about what it's done to me, how it's affected my life. It seems like such a painful way to go about it, though." She was again silent. When she finally spoke, her voice was low, but decisive. "There isn't anything else that we can do then, is there? When do we begin?"

It was only after the session was over and we had spoken of the arrangements concerning the analysis, that I wondered if Ms. B had agreed to the proposed mode of treatment because of an unconscious wish to be punished. As soon as I had the thought, I felt certain of its accuracy. It was obvious enough, and is certainly relevant in the decision to embrace analysis made by most masochistic characters. What I was again uncertain of, however, was the intensity of the unconscious wish to be hurt. Only time would answer the questions my initial sessions with her had posed. Or, more concisely, only a trial of analysis would answer the questions with any degree of accuracy.

A few thoughts concerning my response to the patient seem in order before I describe the analysis itself. I found myself deeply touched by her life story. It had some of the quality of a soap opera, only it had happened to a real person. I realized that I would have to guard against any feelings to want to "make it up to the patient" for her suffering at the hands of others in the past, or to attempt to protect her from future hurt. I also knew that there would be provocations from her that might pull me toward becoming involved with her in a sado-masochistic interaction, with the ultimate aim of actually re-enacting the hurts from the past with me, rather than simply re-experiencing them in the transference.

Another important factor that dictated my decision to suggest analysis to the patient, was her capacity for fantasy. I was in my early forties when I began to treat Ms. B. I had become interested in a group of patients who had a capacity for fantasy and I later wrote about patients who had woven stories about imaginary companions in childhood (Myers, 1976). Some of those patients went on to become writers and artists (see Myers, 1979). Although Ms. B's stories of the adventures with the surrogate parents were not strictly imaginary companion fantasies, they were close enough to attract my interest.

Although such an idiosyncratic interest on the part of the analyst is generally not a good reason for treating a patient analytically, I might note that, in my experience with patients who fantasize imaginary companions in childhood, I had observed that their creations had served to heal narcissistic wounds by erecting idealized self-representations. To state it somewhat differently, the patient's creative adaptation to reality traumata had served her in good stead in the past and had been used to undo the selfsame traumatic experiences she had really experienced. To my mind, this capacity could not help but be useful to her during the periods of transference deprivation in treatment.

When Ms. B first lay down on the couch, she commented on how strange it felt to her to be "lying down on a bed and talking to a man." She half turned around to stare at me several times each session in the first few days of the analysis, as if she were checking to see if I had changed the position of my chair vis-à-vis her. The content of the initial visits dealt somewhat superficially with her pupils and her activities at school. The one or two brief dream fragments offered also dealt with school activities and the patient had few associations to them. Then during a session in the second week of the analysis, she began to cry.

"I just thought about my father," she said, "about his dying and my never getting a chance to really resolve things with him. I never thought he cared at all, until that last conversation. And I never got the opportunity to really know just how much he did."

At the end of this session, she stared at me rather intently as she left the office. When the next session began with a similar stare, and was interspersed with several episodes of turning around to look at me, I asked her about her behavior.

"I don't know why I'm doing it," she said, "it's just as if I have to check that you're not mad at me. Maybe I'm trying to find out from you what I couldn't ever learn from him. I'm not sure."

This early session and her behavior in following sessions could be seen as the beginning of a long period of mourning for the dead father. Many early visits were spent discussing her wishes for what might have been, had he lived. Most of the fantasied talks or trips together, included just the two of them, not the stepmother or stepsisters. Although the implicit content of the fantasies seemed to involve hidden sexual desires toward the father, the predominant explicit content and affect, was with the idea of the loss of the father's ability to love her non-sexually.

During one session in the middle of the third month of the analysis, Ms. B came into the office looking dejected. "I had a bad dream last night," she announced, "about my father. He was at a ceremony, a dedication for a building he had done. The mayor or some other town official had just given a speech honoring my father and then he was introduced as the next speaker. I felt a surge of pride when he got up to talk, but before he could say anything, he just keeled over and was dead. I felt an enormous wave of sadness pass over me and I woke up."

The patient then began to cry. "I don't know why I'm crying now. I mean of course I know, but I just don't understand why all I can think about lately, whenever I come in here, is my father. I realize that the dream is some kind of encapsulated version of what actually happened between the two of us . . . he finally gets ready to talk to me and then he dies. All this feeling that I seem to be dredging up for him . . . it seems so out of proportion to what the actual reality of our lives together consisted of. We barely ever spoke to each other. We drifted through all those years before and after my stepmother came, hardly ever interacting. And now all I can do is cry for him and turn my analysis into some kind of monument to his memory."

When I asked her what her thoughts were about turning the analysis into a monument for her father, she replied: "I haven't been back home in a long time. Not since my little sister got married. And that was a good 15 years ago. But I've been thinking about it a lot recently, about the house we all grew up in. My father designed it and supervised its being built. Come to think of it, it looked a little like the building in the dream. I wish that my stepmother hadn't sold it. I'd like to have it now. The people who bought it redid it so extensively that it barely resembles the original house.

"I know it's supposed to be important for me to talk about my father in here, but I don't really see any good reason for doing that. All I do is get sadder and sadder, when I think about him and what we might have had together. It serves no concrete purpose for me. It's like talking about a ghost, a being with no real structure or substance. It feels false to me, as if I'm constructing some sort of edifice of lies for you. Why do you let me go on wasting my time like this? Why don't you stop me?"

I told her then, that at the selfsame time she was asking me to stop her from talking about her father, her very choice of words and phrases themselves, such as concrete, structure, constructing some sort of edifice, with their obvious identification with her father's architectural pursuits, underscored her conflicting wishes to hang onto him and to continue talking about him. I further observed that the ambivalent attitudes she had now was also depicted in her dream, where the father was first honored and then eliminated. I then questioned her as to whether she had had any specific thoughts about why she wanted me to be the one to decide which of her conflicting desires should be given precedence.

"I wasn't aware that I was doing that," she said softly. "It kind of hurts me to hear you say that, but I think that you're right. I do want you to make the choice and not me."

My later understanding of the patient's being hurt by my intervention involved its activation of two intertwining trends in her character structure, which were to become increasingly manifest as time went on. The first centered about her prominent feelings of guilt, for her libidinal, as well as her aggressive wishes toward her father, and the second dealt with her masochistic feelings toward me in the transference. To either make her continue with the talk about her father, or to allow her to desist, would be tantamount to forcing her to confront the bittersweet feelings of love and loss toward him. But in so forcing her, I would be re-enacting her childhood sado-masochistic relationship to her father. And if I did force her (hurt her or get angry at her), it could be seen as both an expression of my (her father's) love for her and as a justification for her angry feelings to me (him), thereby diminishing her guilt.

Needless to say, I did not interpret my nascent understanding of the intertwining trends to the patient at this point. I was content to let her go on with the flow of her associations.

"I hope you're not mad at me," she said, "I wouldn't like that, if you were. I need to feel that you're on my side, if this is all going to work out. I want to believe that regardless of what I say, you won't be upset by it."

As she spoke, I recognized that she was alluding to an important transference fantasy. The unconscious wish being expressed was that I would be impervious to her anger, unable to be injured or destroyed by it. I was to be different than the father in the dream or the mother, grandmother, or beloved teacher in reality. No matter what, I was to remain alive and also I was not to become angry and retaliate against her or destroy her.

The wish just described above is one of great significance in the treatment of older patients, regardless of the relative importance of their guilt feelings and of the masochistic wishes in their character structure. Since most older individuals suffer some degree of "survivor guilt" vis-à-vis important objects in their life who have died, it is often easier for them to work with a younger analyst or therapist, one they can envision as able to outlive them. This age disparity tends to lead to an overall diminution of the guilt feelings over having survived one's parents, spouse, etc. What must be contended with, however, is the rage toward the younger analyst for his youth, but this can often be more easily dealt with, in my experience, with such patients, than survivor guilt.

"You're right," Ms. B continued, "I want you to be the one to decide if I should talk about my father or not. In one way, it feels good to keep on talking about him, as if I'm close to him in a way that I never was close to him in reality. Only it feels as if there's something wrong with my doing that. Why is it wrong to want to be close to him? Can you explain that to me? I don't understand."

"And if I stop talking about him, it's as if I have to acknowledge that he's dead again. That's so painful. It's almost a matter of it's being in my power to keep him alive by talking about him or to kill him off by letting go of the thoughts about him. It's horrible. I don't want to have to make that kind of decision. It's not fair. Why should I always have to be responsible for every life I come into contact with. I didn't ask for that kind of power. . . ."

Ms. B was silent for several minutes and the session was ending. I thought about questioning her about what she had just said, or perhaps I might point out the implicit wish involved in her musings. She pre-empted my attempt, however, when she noted, "That sounds so crazy, what I was just saying, so godlike of me to say it. My rational side doesn't really believe those ideas, but nonetheless they sometimes feel so very real to me. Rationally, I understand that having the kind of power I was referring to, would have given me a greater degree of control over what happened to me in my life. I could have prevented all of those deaths and not ended up alone and feeling guilty. Help me fight the irrationality in me, please. . . ."

I was touched by this. The clarity of Ms. B's insight and the intensity of her plea for help made me want to protect her. But I said nothing and the session ended.

When the patient returned the next day, she immediately went back to her thoughts about her father. She railed about his death and his abandonment of her, just as she had finally begun to find him. Her anger over the multiple hurts he had inflicted upon her all her life began to emerge in an ever-burgeoning series of temper outbursts. In this session, and in those in the weeks that followed, the saga of her father's "deceits" with the stepmother and with the farm-girl housekeepers was repeated in seemingly endless variations. She raged and stormed at the dead man, in a surprisingly acerbic manner. How could he have hated her? Why was he not the man she had always wished him to be? Why had he sent her off to boarding school? Why had he had any children with her stepmother? Why had he not loved her and known just who she really was? Question followed question and her rising anger knew no bounds.

Interspersed with her outbursts of anger were dramatic periods of weeping. Her sessions were held after school hours and when I once asked her to change the time of a meeting one day to an hour before school, she implored me not to ask, as she could never go to work looking as bad as she did after her visits.

The periodic turning around in sessions to check my expression re-appeared. Visually and verbally, she had to be certain that I was not angry at her for being such an angry person. Surely I had not expected her to be such a "horrible bitch." I must regret my decision to have taken her into analysis. She was sure I would never do it again. Through all this period, I was essentially silent. There was no need to speak and I was quite pleased with the patient's capacity to so express her anger. I had not expected that it would be quite so easy for her.

Shortly before the first summer vacation break in the analysis was to occur, the analytic honeymoon period ended. Ms. B, uncharacteristically, had too much to drink at a party thrown by a colleague at school, and she smashed her car into a stop sign on the highway when she was returning to New York City. Her jaw was broken and one rib was fractured. In addition, her bladder was ruptured and she ended up with peritonitis. The repair of the jaw involved wiring, which necessitated her eating (or, more accurately, drinking) her meals through a straw for a considerable time. All in all, her condition was critical for a week or two and when I was notified, I visited her in the intensive care unit of the hospital before I went on vacation.

A number of thoughts went through my head before I visited the patient. It seemed apparent to me that her sense of guilt over the rage she had been expressing over her father had gotten the best of her. In an economic manner, she had paid the penalty for her crime of rage to the dead parent and enacted her libidinal wish to be close to him by becoming like him. Her drinking had caused an accident that was remarkably similar to the one that had killed her father.

But what seemed to me to be of greater significance was the obvious impetus given to her unconscious need to be punished for the unexpressed anger toward me in the transference. This anger had been aroused because I was leaving on vacation, abandoning her now, as her father had done. I felt guilty at not having interpreted this sufficiently, though I had certainly not let it go by unheeded in the sessions just prior to the accident. I began to wonder if, through some counteridentification with the patient, I was sharing her godlike wish to save the significant others in my life, such as her. At this juncture, I realize that this was one of the important unconscious communications to me involved in the patient's accident, and I decided to interpret this to her when I saw her, if I felt that she was well enough to receive it.

I briefly thought about the breach in strict analytic technique involved in visiting her in the hospital. My concerns, however, were quickly overriden by the gravity of her physical condition and by my fears that she might die. These fears, I might add, were fairly quickly dispelled by her attending physician whom I met as I went in to see Ms. B. He assured me that she was recovering nicely from the peritonitis and from the oral surgery on her jaw. She would do well, he said, but she would probably be in the hospital for a matter of weeks.

I saw my visit to her in the hospital as providing her with a counterpart of the vis-à-vis checks she so often sought in sessions, when she would turn around to study my face. Certainly my visit, and my thinking about her concrete need to see that I was not angry at her, was a parameter in the analysis. In retrospect, I would have surely visited her, if I were to do it over. I am much less certain, however, that I would have felt that she concretely needed to see me in order to check on my response to her self-destructively rageful act.

When I did see her in the hospital, it was very difficult for her to communicate. She was in pain, for one thing, but more significantly, her jaw was wired, so that she had to write her thoughts down. She seemed ill at ease with my visit. For one thing, it was conducted in a vis-à-vis manner, unlike our usual sessions. For another, she was concerned that I would be angry with her for her "stupidity" in having the accident.

"I'm glad you came," she wrote, "but I feel like an ass for the accident. I've never done anything like this before. And I must look a pretty sorry sight right now. There are certain advantages to being on the couch, which I never quite realized till this moment."

As she sipped some water through a bent glass straw, I commented to her that I thought that her accident was connected with the imminence of my departure for my vacation. Her eyes dropped from my face and she sipped intently.

"Aside from feeling guilty at the anger you've been expressing toward your father," I noted, "I think you've also been feeling guilty about the anger you've had toward me because of my going away on vacation. It's another example of the kind of uncontrollable situations which you've been forced to experience all of your life. At some level, I believe that your accident was geared to make me feel the same degree of impotence vis-à-vis my ability to influence you, that you've felt with other people for so many years, and with me about my going on vacation." I was silent and then added: "In addition to wanting to make me feel guilty for what's happened to you, it's as if you don't really believe that what you communicate verbally to me really gets across to me. Somehow you have to show me what you feel through your actions, even if your actions are self-destructive and counter-productive. You don't believe that I'll get what you're trying to communicate to me any other way."

The patient was silent for a long time and I wondered if I had gone too far, as if I had been trying to make up for the flatness of my efforts prior to her accident, in some belated attempt to undo the near-tragedy. Or had I been enacting some sado-masochistic fantasy with her in which I caused her even more pain than she had experienced in the accident? Ms. B then raised her face up from the glass, which had seemed glued to it, and looked directly into my eyes.

"Thank you for coming," she wrote, and the tears streamed down her face. "I don't think that I can digest all that you said right now, but I will think about it before I see you back in the fall." With that, she fleetingly grasped the back of my hand and then lay back down on the bed and closed her eyes. I left the hospital and went on vacation the next day.

When Ms. B returned to the analysis in the fall, she was pale and thin. I had thought about her on a number of occasions while I was away, attempting to understand my concern for her, so that it would not get out of hand and prevent me from making appropriate interpretations. I came to see that my own wishes to protect her from any further hurts in life stemmed, in part, from childhood wishes to be protected from certain hurts I experienced at the hands of my parents. I also felt the need to protect her from my own hostile (sadistic) wishes, which she tended to evoke (and which resonated with the sadistic experiences of her childhood incurred at the hands of her father). What I am noting here is that the masochistic patient often strongly evokes both the wish to hurt and the wish to protect in the analyst, and it is imperative that the analyst understand the roots of these wishes in his own life experiences, if he is not to be drawn into either a sado-masochistic interaction or an overly protective attitude in the transference.

"You really said quite a mouthful to me," Ms. B began, "when you visited me in the hospital. I really am grateful that you came. I kept on thinking there that you wouldn't want to see me after the accident, that you'd blame me and think that I was too sick for the treatment."

Her initial verbalizations tended to corroborate my idea that my visit had served as the equivalent of the movements during sessions, whereby she turned around to check on my expression and my feelings vis-à-vis her. What she said, however, did not answer my question about the necessity of such a visit, because of my fears that she might not be able to handle the intensity of her anger and her guilt feelings.

"It's a lot easier on the couch, than being face to face. I don't think I could talk about all of this, if I were worried about looking at you all of the time. Anyway, I want to go on and talk about a couple of the things that you said to me.

"You didn't mean to imply, did you, that I consciously cracked up my car in order to make you feel guilty about not being able to help me? I hope not, because I certainly had no conscious awareness of that when I left the party. If you're talking about my unconscious, I can't answer for that directly, but you might be right. I was mad at you for leaving me, madder than I could acknowledge to myself at that time. It seemed cruel to me, after all I'd been saying for so long about my father. It still does. As if you're just as uncaring a person as he was, and haven't really been listening to me at all. As if you don't give a damn, just like him. I know that's not really true. You did come to the hospital. But you never called me after that to ask me how I was doing. That bothered me. I still feel hurt by it." At this point, Ms. B began to cry.

Somewhere during the course of her speech, I realized the truth involved in the principle of deprivation in analysis. No matter what I might have wanted to give the patient to make up for her childhood deprivations, it would never have been enough. The only approach that would be of any real help to her in the long run would be an analysis of her feelings about the childhood situation, as re-directed toward me in the analytic transference. Moreover, I perceived her anger toward me at that moment as verifying of the truth of my earlier interpretations to her. If anything, she was continuing in her attempt to make me feel impotent vis-à-vis her.

Once more, Ms. B seemed to divine my thoughts and to preempt my interpretation. "I suppose you're going to say," she observed, "that I'm still trying to make you feel guilty right now, when I criticized you for not calling me over the summer. You're really pretty self-centered, if you think that. Not every action that I perform in my life revolves around you. It makes me mad to think that you believe that it does. You may be right, though, when you say I'm not so sure that what I tell you really gets across to you. I don't see how it can. If it did, you would have checked up on me and not let me go the whole month without my hearing from you."

The intensity of Ms. B's anger surprised me and caught me off guard. I recognized, however, that she was able to express her anger so intensely because her superego had been mollified by the accident itself. As a result of her suffering, she had temporarily paid her dues and could justify her outburst.

The barrage of anger and the perception of me as cold and ungiving, much in the manner of the abandoning father, persisted for many months during the second year of analysis. I was told that my interpretations were intellectual and not feeling or that I was an intelligent automaton, programmed to receive data and to respond mechanically. She wondered why she was in analysis, as things did not seem to be changing in her life. If anything, they were getting worse, not better. She barely had any interest in her own photography anymore and she had no interest in seeing friends or in doing anything socially. If the analysis was supposed to help her get closer to men, it certainly wasn't doing that, because she hadn't even started to date, let alone begun to deal with her sexual hangups.

During this long siege of rage toward me in the transference, my only real concern was that she not pay too high a price for it, because of her masochistic character structure. The blunting of the pleasure she derived from her artistic activities and the social withdrawal seemed to be sufficient to balance the books over the expression of her rage to me. I kept hoping that no greater price than that would be exacted by her superego for her anger.

Because of Ms. B's response to my prior vacation, I was concerned over what might happen when I left for a brief spring holiday. I expended a considerable amount of effort beforehand on interpreting whatever connections became apparent between her anger and my impending vacation. She would often agree with what I had said, and then would berate me for leaving her once more, for being just like all of the people who had left her in the past.

"It wouldn't matter to you if I were dead when you got back," Ms. B announced near the beginning of the session before my departure.

"Is it really necessary that you punish yourself so severely," I asked, "for the anger you feel at my leaving? I understand that you feel that I'm killing you, when I go away, but is it essential to really do it to yourself in order to make me believe how you feel?"

"There you go again with interpretation number seven. The patient doesn't feel that the doctor understands her when she speaks to him, so she has to convey her feelings through the desperateness of her actions. Right out of the textbook, doctor, or is it the computer?"

I felt frustrated; it was difficult dealing with a patient who was essentially trying to blackmail me emotionally. She had succeeded in raising the level of my anxiety about leaving her. Other patients often made comments, or even threats, about what might befall them when I was away, but those utterances rarely had to be given much credence. A variety of speeches about my not being able to conduct an analysis under the threat of blackmail crossed my mind, but I did not make them. Instead, I noted:

"I wonder if what's going on with us now is really an example of the extraordinary sensitivity to feeling slighted, which you've suffered from all of your life. You've had a lot of real hurts and real slights in your life, and they've sensitized you to perceiving hurts and slights in situations where the issues aren't quite the same. Yes, I am leaving now and I know that hurts you. But that isn't quite the same as saying that I planned this trip in order to hurt you. It's that distinction which seems to be so difficult for you to see.

"Further, I recognize that not being able to get me to change my mind about going away does make you feel exceptionally powerless and that's a very lousy feeling to have. Though it is a familiar one for you. But I'm not going away specifically in order to make you feel powerless and I do hope that you are able to see that idea."

Ms. B was silent for a long period of time and I wondered if my words had had any impact at all. I became even more concerned about what might happen to her when I was away. I also began to seriously second guess myself about the correctness of choosing analysis for her. It struck me, then, that I had drastically underestimated the intensity of her masochism.

"You know," she said, "I have the impression for the first time in a long time, that you really do care. But there's something you still don't understand about all of this. Intellectually, I know that what you're saying is true. I am extrasensitive to feeling hurt. The antennae are always out there to pick up the slings and arrows that come my way. But my 'paranoia' about being specially singled out to be slighted has its positive features, too. At least that way, I know that I count. You just told me that you're not going away specifically to make me feel powerless. But don't you see that it might be better, from my point of view, if you were. I'd have to mean an awful lot to you, for you to single me out so vindictively. And that's the very least that I deserve. It's not being special that drives me up a wall. All the pain and suffering in my life has got to have made me special. And if you take that away from me, it's tantamount to my not amounting to anything at all. I won't let you do that to me. Do you understand?"

And I did understand what she meant. She had just offered to me a clear-cut exposition of the psychology of the exception. By virtue of the early and ongoing suffering in her life, she believed that she deserved to be treated as special. What was curious about Ms. B was that she had never carried this idea to its usual extreme. Most individuals who are driven by this type of unconscious fantasy, generally rebel. They have a sense of entitlement, which allows them to contravene the usual rules of society, such as the oedipal injunctions. Ms. B, however, was unable to live out the excesses justified by the fantasy. She did not sleep with the teacher's husband, for example, whereas the usual "exception" might have. Unfortunately, I have no ready explanation to offer for the restraints shown by my patient in this area.

When I responded to Ms. B, all I said was "I really do understand what you're saying."

She turned her head to look at me and I stared intently into her eyes. The interaction certainly constituted a mini-parameter in the analysis, but this time I felt that it was a necessary one. Perhaps I was acknowledging her "specialness" at that moment, by not attempting to analyze the gesture. Be that as it may, she nodded her head at me in assent, and I felt freer than I had felt all session about the prospect of leaving to go on vacation.

"Have a good trip," she said, as she came to the door.

"Thanks," I responded, and smiled at her.

When I returned from the trip, her anger was still apparent but muted. The visual checking was also intermittently present over the first week or two after my return, then it disappeared for a long while. I was surprised when she reported having actually taken some photographs during my absence. She had not done this for many months.

About a month after my return from the spring trip, Ms. B dreamt about being in a sensual embrace with a man. His features were indeterminate in the dream, but the patient described the curious sensation of feeling his glasses in the breast pocket of his jacket, as her body was crushed up against his.

"One of the teachers in my school keeps his glasses there," she noted. "He's quite an attractive man. We were talking about photography last week and I noticed them in there. He's a science teacher. Funny thing, L [her mentor's husband] was a science teacher, too."

She hesitated at this point, and I asked her what she was thinking about.

"I was thinking about the sexual feelings in the dream. I think about that time with L whenever I feel sexy. It felt good in the dream, being pressed up against his body like that."

The patient squirmed and twisted on the couch and tried to turn her face and body away from me, so that I could not look at her. She seemed unable to continue. I simply commented on the fact that she seemed uncomfortable about my being able to see her face and body.

"I'm ashamed of what you'll see. As if you can tell how hot I feel from the way I look. I wonder what would have happened to my life, if I had slept with L? Would it really have changed things? How different would I be right now?"

When the session ended, Ms. B blushed as she walked past me to the door of my office. She turned her face from mine and tried to draw her body in upon itself, as if to defend herself from my gaze.

"I didn't want to tell you," she said the next day, "but I've seen you carrying your glasses in your jacket pocket, at times. Oh God, I can't go on with this now. It's too embarrassing."

She did go on, however, and in a session a few days later, she revealed that she had masturbated for the first time in a long while with the fantasy of being pressed up against me. Over the next few months, the man with the glasses became the prototype of her masturbatory fantasies. Many of these directly involved me, as she had mentioned. Others dealt with her mentor's husband, L, and still others dealt with the science teacher and with other men at her school.

For a long time, she was inhibited in talking about the details of the fantasies. She described them in vague terms, and only in response to a direct question, would she acknowledge that the fantasies and the masturbation culminated in an orgastic release. One day, I inquired further about the curious detail of the glasses.

Ms. B blushed once more and drew up into herself again. "I don't like to talk about that," she said. "It makes me feel like a freak of some kind."

After a considerable period of hemming and hawing, she finally admitted that in some of her fantasies, the man would look at her naked body with his glasses on. "I feel terrible talking about this," she murmured. "I don't want you to look at me now. Oh what am I saying? I do want you to look, yes I do." With this, she began to cry. "It's too difficult to talk about it, because it makes me want it right now, to have you look at me."

Shortly before the second summer vacation break, we began to understand more about the man in the glasses theme. Ms. B recalled that her father had kept a magnifying glass on his desk. He would check details on his plans with it, to make certain that they were correct. She remembered that on certain occasions, she would use the magnifying glass to study anatomical drawings in an encyclopedia her father kept in his bedroom. Thus, the study of male and female anatomical differences became associated in her mind with the use of a glass (glasses) and was connected with her father's bedroom. When I inquired as to whether she had ever seen or heard her father and stepmother in bed together, she answered that she could not recall. She did remember seeing her father with some of the farm-girl housekeepers, however, and she was then able to recall how angry he had been when he saw her standing in the doorway observing him in bed with a young woman.

"His eyes seemed all contorted then," she noted, "as if they were about to pop out of his head. It was probably just his response at being discovered by me, but it scared me and made a deep impression on me."

I commented to her that her fantasy of the man with the glasses seemed to have a number of determinants, all centering on the themes of looking at someone sexually or being looked at in a sexual way. I suggested that she had been aroused, as well as frightened, as a child, by seeing her father with a young woman, and that she had wished to be the one in bed with him. She blushed again, when I said this, but did not rebut my comments. I further observed that she must have wondered about what her beloved teacher and her husband did in bed together and perhaps her thoughts about them had further aroused her.

"I saw them having intercourse one time," she said, interrupting me. "They didn't know I was there. It was that summer that we all spent together. I was supposed to be out for a walk and they must have thought that they were in the house alone. I never told them that I saw them. I was just walking by their bedroom and the door was open, when I think I heard them first and I stopped walking. Then I sort of peered in and peeked at them. They never knew. You're right, though, I did think about that a lot and it did arouse me. I wanted L a lot, I think. Sometimes I'd go over to see her, just in order to be around him. It was so hard to admit that to myself. I felt so ungrateful for having those desires, after all she'd done for me. In some of the daydreams I had during my 'teen years, I'd think of us all coming down to New York City and then some of the art would get lost and L would take me with him to look for it. And we would get caught in the rain and have to change our clothes and he'd look at me. Oh God, it's hard to talk about this. When he finally did kiss me that time, I wanted him so badly that I guess I didn't know what to do. But I felt so guilty. She was barely dead, and she'd been so good to me. I think I felt angry at him because it was like his making me choose between the two of them and I couldn't do that then."

She cried deeply then, but was able to acknowledge that she had also thought about my wife a good deal and wondered just what she was like. She imagined that we would spend a lot of time together in bed during our vacation and she grudgingly admitted that she would like to be the one there. With this updated transference version of the oedipal fantasy of the man with the glasses, the second year of the analysis came to an end. Very little of the anger that had characterized the first year and one-half of treatment was still apparent in the sessions just before the vacation break. And this time I was able to leave without feeling apprehensive about what might happen to her during my absence.

When I returned in the fall, I was surprised when she did not appear for her first two sessions. I became concerned and then she appeared the third day at her appointed hour. "I wasn't sure if I wanted to come back in," she said. "I've been very upset while you were away. I thought things'd be all right when you left, but they weren't. I had a date with the science teacher at school and it was a disaster. He tried to kiss me and I practically had a fit. I didn't know whether to run away or to smash his teeth in. I never realized that I had so much anger to men. You shouldn't have let me get into a situation like that. I felt like a fool. I'll never be able to look him in the eye again at school."

I thought that the theme of looking and being looked at had not diminished over the summer holiday break. Certainly the date with the science teacher had been a response to her feelings of abandonment by me in the transference. But it was a rotten piece of luck, I thought, that it had gone so poorly. I suggested to Ms. B that some of the anger she had felt toward the teacher must have been aroused by the idea of my having left her to be with my wife. I further wondered with her if she had any ideas about why she had felt so frightened about the encounter. Why had she wanted to run away from him?

"There you go again," she said, "all you ever care about is trying to analyze things. Why don't you try to put yourself in my shoes and imagine how I felt when it happened and not worry about why it happened? I made a fool of myself. Doesn't that register with you at all? Don't you care about the fact that you left me alone and gave me carte blanche to go ahead with things and I made a mess of them? I wasn't ready for it. Maybe I never will be. You should have known better. You should have seen that and warned me about what was going to happen."

The theme of my being a bad parent who was unresponsive to her needs and who allowed her to expose herself to dangerous situations arose in session after session. Again she withdrew socially and stopped taking photographs. She spoke about these issues in terms of vindictively wanting to deprive me of my chance to achieve any analytic success with her, as well as in terms of her own inadequacy and unworthiness. Whatever I said to her seemed to be wrong. I was either too mechanical, too intellectual, too robotic, or too analytic. The theme of the man with the glasses had long since disappeared from view, as had any mention of masturbatory fantasies. We seemed enmeshed in her transference rage at me for being the unprotecting parent.

It slowly became clear that the major focus of the patient's rage was upon the issue of my not having prepared her to deal adequately with a man. I had not taught her the finer points of making small talk or the nuances of kissing and petting. And anything beyond that was a total mystery. How could I let my analytic offspring risk so much, when she was so ill equipped and ill prepared?

As I listened to the litany of complaints against me, session after session, I began to think of them in terms of an adolescent girl's polemic against a mother who has not prepared her for her role as a woman. The intrinsic logic of the patient's complaints inevitably began to strike me as so obvious that I wondered why I had taken so long to come to this realization. Finally, I began to interpret some of these issues to the patient.

I told her that her complaints against me had the ring of a girl's cries against an inadequate or absent mother, something which Ms. B had obviously good cause to rail against. First her own mother had died, and then her grandmother. The farm-girl housekeepers were hardly an able lot and her stepmother was, at best, an indifferent participant in her life. The only good woman she had ever really known had been her teacher, and though she had helped the patient to attain an understanding of art and poetry, she had not imparted much fundamental sexual information to her beyond explaining the menarche. These comments were followed by a storm of long pent-up anger from the patient, directed toward the formerly hallowed teacher.

"How could she not talk to me about anything else beside my periods? Where did she think that I was going to learn that stuff from?"

I might note here, that the patient had actually learned about conception from one of the maids in the house. And she had talked a little with her classmates in school about kissing and petting and sexual relationships. So although her complaints were true, overall, the exceptions to the rule belied their global validity.

Throughout the third year of the analysis, the one constant theme was this issue of the missing mother. The lamentations for the dead father, which had played such an important part in the early days of analysis, were replaced by the even more poignant grieving for the lost mother. In dream after dream, the patient portrayed a madonna-like version of the mother. In other instances, the colors in the dreams seemed to be the carriers of the affective charges, as when a dream of union with the mother took place in a proverbial scene of green pastures or another dream involving the mother's loss was represented in somber hues of deep blues and blacks.

Alternating with the grieving for the dead idealized mother, were the equally intense storms of rage at the mother, now devalued. She was seen as worthless or was portrayed in dreams as a decayed corpse covered with maggots or as a hapless cretin. When I went off on my usual spring holiday, I was once more blasted for my unreliability and my inadequacy. I was, clearly now, the hapless mother, devalued and denigrated to insignificance. What was the point of the treatment, she wondered? What could someone as young and untalented as I was offer her? Maybe we should reverse roles. Maybe she should be the analyst and the mother. She would know how to do it right. All she would have to do would be to plumb the depths of her own experience, to find out how to help her patients. She would be the better analyst.

My interpretations about her wish to assume my analytic functions in order to allay her feelings of loss over the period of separation (an identification with the abandoning aggressor analyst) fell on deaf ears. I was being too mechanical and too robotic and too intellectual. She had warmth, I was totally devoid of it. My wife could have me, I was probably a lousy lover anyway. In this setting, I noted that she was also describing me frequently as being emasculated. I was seen as either a castrated male or an aphallic mother. In any event, I was hardly capable of offering her a phallus or its equivalent in fantasy. I pointed out that she had spoken of me as a eunuchoid figure, incapable of offering her the strength she wished for in her interactions with people.

"You're right," she said, "I do see you that way. And what good are you for me like that. You're not a strong enough man to either make me into a real woman or to impart your masculinity to me so that I don't have to deal with that issue at all. It's easier to be a man. And a lot safer, too. You don't have to worry about getting pregnant and dying, like my mother did." Here the patient began to weep again and to once more re-experience the loss of the dead mother and the mother surrogates. "Damn my father," she continued, "he should have been the one to die first, instead of her!"

After my return from the vacation trip, she continued railing at me for not being an adequate man. Alternating with her denigrating comments about my masculinity, were her fantasies of what it would have been like for her to have been born a boy.

"My father would have loved me," she mused. "I could have gone into his firm with him and we could have built houses together. I could have had a lot of lovers, those girls he slept with seemed so easy. I could have even had. . . ."

When she hesitated, I waited a moment and then she supplied the ending to the sentence "my teacher." After a momentary silence, Ms. B tentatively continued. "Does that make me homosexual? I did want her or something like that. In some of the daydreams when L and I got caught in the rain, she'd be there, too, and we'd all have to change our clothes together. He'd look at us and I'd look at them. His big penis scared me. It really did, that time I saw them. Her breasts were sweet and small. They seemed natural. I don't like talking about this. It makes me feel so odd, so distant."

In the sessions before the summer break, the oddness and distance seemed to grow. There was a vague feeling of uncertainty and disconnection in the transference relationship, as if Ms. B's anger toward me was threatening to get the better of the bond between us. On my return in the fall, I half expected that she might miss one or two of the early sessions, as she had done the year before. Instead, she arrived early for the first session we had scheduled and smiled cryptically at me, as she entered by office.

"It's been quite a summer," she announced, "quite a summer indeed! I finally slept with someone."

I was startled by this piece of unexpected "good news." It was the last thing I had anticipated, considering the sessions prior to my departure. Perhaps I had misjudged the strength of the transference relationship, I thought. It must not have been precarious as I had felt it to be.

"Her name is Ellen," Ms. B continued, interrupting my self-congratulatory reverie. "We met at the inn that I was staying at in New England."

In her characteristic manner, the patient managed to immediately divine my consternation. She turned around quite suddenly to look at me, after her announcement, and managed to observe my facial expression as my face dropped in open-mouthed amazement. The hostility evident in her sardonic smile was quite apparent, but it seemed mixed with something else, which I was unable to discern then. For a brief while, it seemed as if the previous three years had gone for naught, as if there had been no alliance between us.

I was aware of feeling quite deflated, and then the images floating through my mind struck a familiar chord. The summer absence had obviously been undone by the relationship, and the theme of the missing mother had been fused with that of the missing phallus. Only this time, the phallus that was supposed to be missing was my own. Obviously Ms. B had chosen the single most telling blow she could imagine to strike at my sense of myself as an effective analyst and man. How she had managed to recognize my investment in her achieving heterosexual pleasure so accurately, was hard for me to comprehend, but she had. She had somehow intuited my periodic departures from the stance of analytic neutrality in this area, and she had engineered my "come uppance" in the most "castrating" manner she could think of. Needless to say, there were many determinants in her choice of a woman as a lover. Of paramount significance, however, was its value as a means of expressing her castrating rage toward me for my paternal abandonment of her in the summer vacations and my transference incapacity in the three prior years of the analysis to make up for her past deprivations.

I said nothing for a while, and the patient went on to describe the manner of her meeting with Ellen and some of the nuances of their relationship. She even volunteered some of the details of their sexual interactions, which largely consisted of kissing, cuddling, and mutual masturbatory play to orgasm. As she went on with her "victory" speech, the pleasurable quality in her voice began to disappear and it became monotonous. Suddenly, she was the one who appeared deflated, as if she had just perceived that her triumph over me was a pyrrhic one. She fell silent then and quiet tears slowly dripped down her cheeks.

"Perhaps you're not as angry at me as you thought you were," I noted softly, "or the victory's not as sweet as you expected it to be. I sense that you wanted to prove that you could make me feel as poorly about myself as you've so often felt about yourself. Only to reduce me and emasculate me, doesn't elevate and endow you in quite the way you hoped it would. If anything, you seem to be feeling guilty about it now and rather depressed. If I get pushed down to the bottom of the scrap heap, then there isn't anyone out here at all to help you. So it's better to have the blind leading the blind, so to speak, than to have no one there at all."

Ms. B briefly spoke of how Ellen was able to do this for her now, but her crying grew more vocal and continued till the end of the session and throughout the better part of the next few sessions. At moments, she would defiantly continue to espouse the validity of and the sexual gratifications inherent in the relationship with Ellen. But her anger seemed muted and aborted, as if she had run out of steam. This liaison itself, however, continued, month after month, and I began to realize that there were really many positive features in the interaction between the two women. It was quite apparent that they cared a great deal about each other and met many of their mutual reality needs. Sexually, the interaction was very enjoyable for both of them and none of the anger and the fear that had marked Ms. B's episode with the male science teacher marred their union.

Although an important aspect of the patient's relationship with Ellen represented an acting out of aspects of the transference, which was the initial focus of my interpretative interventions, as time went on the reality elements became of increasing significance in the overall assessment of the situation. Ms. B became increasingly able to acknowledge her castrative rage to me and to her father, as well as her terrifying fears of being damaged (torn apart) in sexual relations with a man. Her wishes for union with the dead mother–grandmother–stepmother–teacher, were also more frequently verbalized and were related to the gratifications inherent in the liaison with Ellen. She seemed happier and a considerable amount of new material about her early years with the grandmother and with the farm-girl housekeepers began to emerge. She even expressed feelings of warmth to me, wishing me well and telling me that she would miss me when I went on a spring vacation, in words without the usual anger and guilt-engendering provocativeness. Without question, she was a lot easier to work with than she had been in the past. But I began to feel that something of the "heart and soul" of the treatment seemed to have disappeared. It lacked the intensity in the transference that it had had in the past, and I was uncertain if this depth of feeling would ever return.

When we resumed the analysis after my holiday, Ms. B told me that she was seriously considering terminating the analysis when we reached the summer break. The news did not surprise me. Once more, I suggested that her statement could be seen as an obvious form of retaliation for my having just been away.

"I don't think so," she said, "I think I'm past that kind of thing. I genuinely care for you, you know. And my caring transcends my anxieties and my petty vindictiveness. Or maybe it's not so petty. Anyway, you've stood by me through an incredible amount of abuse. I don't know anyone else who would have taken that much shit from me. I don't even know if Ellen would have done that for me. Fortunately, I haven't felt the kind of anger toward her that I felt for you, so I've never had to test out her ability to withstand it. I think she would be able to deal with it, though, no matter what."

"I'm not quite sure I understand then, why you want to stop the analysis," I responded. "Can you tell me what your thoughts are about it?"

"I think I've gone about as far as I can go. I'm sure if I persisted, I would dredge up more memories about my childhood, but they'd only be icing on the cake. I know it was a terrible time. In reality, I've come to understand about my past and to pretty much forgive my father and my mother. And that's what really counts, not all the myriad details of the day-to-day disasters.

"I don't know whether I could sleep with a man now or not. I might still be too frightened. I'm not really sure. I don't think it makes an awful lot of difference whether I'm with a man or a woman. What does matter is that I'm with someone. I actually do like men now, and I've learned to like them by learning to like you, in spite of my anger toward you. You've got your failings, your little pomposities, but basically, you're a nice person and you do care about me. And I'm glad that you were my analyst. Because you taught me how to care, too."

Despite my repeated interpretive efforts about her having to be the one to do the leaving, rather than dealing with her anxieties about being left, or my attempts to probe further into her fear of men, Ms. B persisted in her decision to terminate the analysis by the summer break, at the end of the fourth year of the treatment. Dreams of my death, and of her parents' deaths, emerged during the ensuing months, and she expressed a great deal of sadness at the idea of not seeing me. She could intellectually acknowledge that my comments about her leaving me in order to save me (the continuation of the Typhoid Mary thesis concerning the effects of her anger upon those close to her) might be true, but she still wanted to stop the treatment. She spoke of having to go on with her life and of the need to break the ties with me, so that she could more fully involve herself with Ellen.

She finally tendered her resignation to the school system. She and Ellen traveled to another state and found a charming area where they could set up housekeeping and pursue their mutual interests. When the patient came for her last session, she asked me whether she could sit in the chair that final day. She spoke of wanting to leave me on an equal footing. I concurred with her request.

"If I ever need you again," she asked, "can I come back? You'll be here, won't you?"

"Of course," I answered. "You can always come back whenever you need to."

She chatted on about her plans for a while. And then she said: "You're really all the people I've lost in my life rolled up into one. My mother, my father, my teacher, everyone. Ellen doesn't really feel that way to me, right now. She feels like someone totally new, without the baggage from the past. I want to keep her that way. I think you're right, though, about my having to be the one to do the leaving, rather than risk being left. I couldn't stand to have that happen to me again."

As Ms. B said all of this, she looked at me quite directly, in a vestige of the old checking mechanisms from the past. I responded to this quite simply. "I understand," I said, "it's all right with me." She then stood up and shook my hand and left the office.

In looking back at some of the important features of Ms. B's analysis, a number of things stand out. Obviously, the treatment was aborted prematurely; it was incomplete. This was not a function of the patient's age, however, but rather a function of the scars left by her early and ongoing traumata. Her masochistic character structure posed difficulties for the analysis, but these difficulties would have been encountered at any age period in her life, and certainly were not clearly related to her being over 50 when she started the treatment.

To say that the analysis was an unfinished one because she did not achieve heterosexuality, is, I believe, a limited way of conceptualizing it. More to the point is that a woman with limited object-relationships throughout her life achieved a deep and satisfactory relationship with another person, including a gratifying sexual interaction. That this other person happened to be another woman was perhaps more than simply incidental, but it is not crucial to whether or not the treatment was successful in achieving its major goals. Her rage to both men and women was dramatically muted, as was her fear of closeness. Her need to punish herself was also considerably lessened. She had successfully grieved for the important love objects in her life, including the analyst. In addition, she had found a satisfying career to pursue in her older years in a location that resembled the town of her birth. In other words, she could go home again, without significant guilt or rage or pain. From my point of view, these achievements add up to a major success story, even without the realization of heterosexuality.

5
THERAPY OF A DEPRESSED MAN: Mr. W

Mr. W was referred to me at the age of 62 by his internist, who felt he was depressed and needed treatment. "I'm at a loss as to what to do," the patient announced, "all of the stabilizers I've had in life are gone. My wife, my health, my business, they've all evaporated into thin air. I don't know what's left for me now. I see the kids, but even that doesn't feel solid to me. Everything I've built up seems so ephemeral, as if it's all some sleight of hand trick that's about to come down around my ears."

The patient had been out of work since his company went bankrupt, some four years earlier. A marketing executive, he had managed a major division in his firm. He had always thought of himself as a capable businessman, but since the debacle in his company, he felt uncertain about his skills, despite having attained a considerable degree of financial security through sound investments. This uncertainty about his viability in the job market had been accentuated for him by the fact that he had had no job offers (nor had he solicited any) in the past four years and none seemed to be forthcoming.

Three years before his referral, Mr. W had been awakened in the middle of the night by a crushing chest pain. Rushed to the hospital, he was diagnosed as suffering an acute myocardial infarction. Even though the attack had been relatively mild, and the limitations on his life were negligible, the specter of the attack hung like a Damoclean sword over his head. He found it difficult to verbalize his anxieties about his life and his feelings of inadequacy as a man to his wife, and had gradually withdrawn from their sexual relationships. Despite his subliminal perception of his rejection of his wife, in this regard, he was shocked when she informed him that she was leaving him. This occurred some two years before he first saw me in consultation. He was even more astonished to discover that she had formed an intimate liaison with one of their close friends. He began to think everything and everyone about him untrustworthy. Mr. W sensed a grayness hanging over his world, although he noted that he could have easily lifted it by taking an interest in something.

In the two years since his wife left him, the patient had gone out with only a few women. He found himself going through the motions in conversations and he could not wait to take them home. Sexual approaches seemed out of the question. Besides, he felt no real stirring toward these women and had to acknowledge that he was still tied to his wife by the bonds of a 35-year-old marriage. There was deep hurt in his voice when he spoke of his former wife, however, for she had refused his pleas for a reconciliation when she left him. She had even informed him, to his chagrin and humiliation, that their lovemaking had never been to her liking, as she felt that he had never really considered her satisfaction and gratification.

Mr. W's two children lived at a considerable distance from New York. His son, aged 33, lived in a far Western state with his wife and two children. His 31-year-old daughter lived in the deep south with her husband and three sons. Both children asked Mr. W to spend time with them, which he did, but despite their kindness and concern, he felt "out of synch" with them. He attributed this to his general depression and malaise. He also wondered if the generation gap had managed to isolate him from his progeny. Although he telephoned them weekly, and although his daughter, in particular, sent him special cards and thoughtful gifts, these contacts seemed to lack the real pleasure they had had for him in the past.

In spite of his depression, Mr. W had no real sleep difficulty and his appetite remained good, as did his energy level. He joined a gym and jogged with some enthusiasm. Since his coronary, he had not had further chest pains and the only reminders of the attack were occasional anxiety dreams in which he relived that terrifying night. These nightmares, themselves, had diminished in frequency in the two months before he came to see me.

Mr. W was born in New York City to an upper-middle-class WASP family. His father, an alumnus of an Ivy League college, was a senior officer in one of the large city banks. His mother was a graduate of a select eastern women's school. Both his parents were involved in a variety of civic and charitable pursuits and athletic endeavors. The patient was the eldest of three children, with a sister being born when he was aged two and one-half and a brother when he was five.

Mr. W's parents were hardly neglectful of their children, inasmuch as they were genuinely interested in their progress in school and in their extracurricular activities. Neither one, however, was given to displays of physical affection. To an outside observer, the three siblings would have appeared to have been close to each other, with an evident concern for the others' well-being, but they were always reserved and rarely interacted physically. Little of the usual sibling horseplay took place in Mr. W's household, despite the general interest in athletics. Whatever the hostility, it was usually verbal.

The patient did well at one of the better private schools for boys in the city. He was also a good athlete, but he preferred individual sports, such as track and tennis, rather than such team sports as football or basketball, in which physical contact was an important part of the game. Although he had some friends at school, there was never anyone with whom he was especially close. When it came time to go to boarding school, he was not enthusiastic about leaving home. He knew, however, that he would have to, as it was expected of him.

When he actually went off to boarding school, he was acutely homesick for the first few weeks. He desperately longed to see his brother and sister and to hear their sniping jokes around the family dinner table. He gradually made friends with some of his classmates, however, and was able to overcome his longing for his family. His intelligence and his modest athletic achievements also brought him a degree of admiration from his peers and teachers, which helped make up for the sense of separation he felt from his family. And when he felt overwhelmed, he daydreamed about the good times he had spent fishing with his father in the Canadian woods.

When he graduated from boarding school, Mr. W went to the Ivy League college his father had attended. He joined many of the same clubs, took many of the same courses, and achieved approximately the same degree of academic success. When one of the professors praised his writing ability, he briefly toyed with the idea of becoming a novelist, but he soon dropped it and decided to obtain a master's degree in business administration, as his father had done. On the day of his graduation from business school, Mr. W's father shook his son's hand warmly and told him how proud he was of him and his achievements. The patient reveled in this veritable "orgy" of paternal praise and considered the day one of the highpoints of his life. The year was 1941, and the war in Europe seemed of little relevance to the graduate. America was finally coming out of the Great Depression and the patient later recollected that the idea of the world being his oyster had crossed his mind that day. He did not connect, at the time, his heady state of mind and the obvious approval of both his parents.

Through one of his father's friends, Mr. W obtained a job at an old-line investment banking firm on Wall Street. He tried to throw himself into his work with the same abandon and sense of exhilaration as some of his peers, but he felt uncomfortable with the impersonality at the firm. He never voiced his concerns, however, for he was confident that he would overcome them, as he had overcome his loneliness at boarding school. He also did not wish to displeasure his father or undo any of the sense of closeness he had felt on his graduation from business school.

Fortunately for Mr. W, the war intervened, and when the Japanese attacked Pearl Harbor, it seemed like a deus ex machina to him, rescuing him from his job. He obtained a commission in the Army Air Force and was sent for fighter pilot training. He did reasonably well, as it fit in with his penchant for individual sports. The men he flew with seemed quite different than his Ivy League and Wall Street chums. They came from all walks of life and from many different parts of the country. Most of them seemed more extroverted and more given to a kind of braggadocio his father would have frowned upon. He liked them, however, and this both surprised and worried him. It seemed once more as if something had separated him from his family. Only this time, he felt it was not only a physical distance, but also a difference in values.

During his months in flight school in an air base in the South, the patient chanced to run into a college classmate who lived in the small city near the base. The other man introduced the patient to his sister and the two of them quickly began "keeping company." Although the patient knew that the young woman's family background and social credentials were impeccable, he was worried that his parents might disapprove of her because he had found her himself and not through the social channels he would have gone through had he still lived in New York.

When Mr. W finished flight school, his parents attended his graduation ceremony, where the patient introduced them to his sweetheart. They seemed pleased with her, but he felt disappointed when they simply kissed the young woman on the cheek, rather than warmly embracing her, as he had seen other parents do with young women in similar situations. He was even more upset when his parents disapproved of his desire to marry immediately. For perhaps the first time in his life, he stood his ground and they agreed. The wedding took place in 1943, shortly before the patient was shipped overseas to England.

In England, Mr. W flew fighter support for bomber raids, in the softening-up process prior to D-Day. His plane was the P-51 Mustang, a dangerous but efficient machine, which he maneuvered skillfully. Although he never shirked his duties, and he was in combat on a great number of occasions, he lacked the daredevil qualities of so many of his comrades. He was a "solid" pilot and a sober citizen, fun to be with, but never "outrageous" or "wacky," as some of the other men were. He registered three "kills" in combat, although he did not seem especially proud of the achievement, feeling that he should have done more. After all, it took five "kills" to be an "ace," and his father would have been prouder of him if he had become an ace. Because of his sobriety and caution, he became the paragon of longevity in his squadron. He outlived the more daring fliers, and the more realistic of his squadron mates sought him as a "wing man," thinking him lucky. In two years, he flew one hundred combat missions. His life was endangered on only one occasion, when a stray flak burst damaged his horizontal stabilizer and he was forced down in the English Channel, where he was quickly pulled out of the water by a friendly patrol boat.

When the war ended in Europe, Mr. W was not transferred to

the Pacific theatre of operations, as so many of his fellow fliers were. He remained on at headquarters on a special assignment. One of the generals there knew the patient's father and remembered the young man from a dinner at the family home. Also, the general was interested in having the patient remain in the service after the war. He had heard of Mr. W's special skills at staying alive and his record for caution and sobreity.

"You're the kind of man that we need as an example for the younger pilots coming in," the general said, "not the headline jockeys we've been promoting so hard in the papers." Although the general's offer was flattering, there was something in it that seemed at odds with the patient's sense of himself as a man. He also wanted to be away from war, and back home with his wife, in a job that utilized his talents better than his previous one. What never crossed his mind was the fact that, for the second time in recent years, he had stood up to a paternal figure and insisted on his own desires and his own goals in life.

Shortly after the patient returned to New York and left the service, his wife V became pregnant. A son was born in 1945, a few months after Mr. W entered the company he was to remain with for the next 30 years. The firm, a family business, was run by two brothers. One of the founding fathers had a son, G, who had been a pilot with the patient in England during the war and who had suggested to his father that Mr. W join the company. Both partners liked the young man, and he liked them. The partners seemed interested in what he thought on various matters, and they had an easygoing conversational style, occasionally laced with profanity and off-color jokes, that differed markedly from that of the patient's father. They also were not averse to putting their arms about the shoulders of the young man, showing the warmth they felt toward him. Mr. W knew that his father would have preferred that he return to a career in banking, but the company he was working for was solid, and his father never criticized the patient's choice.

Two years after his son was born, the patient's wife bore him a daughter. The family settled into a pleasant enough life-style, living in the city during the year and spending summers in Maine with the children and with some executives from the patient's company, who became close personal friends. Mr. W enjoyed becoming more his own man. He maintained cordial ties with his parents and was deeply upset when first his mother and then his father passed away when he was in his early forties. The deaths of his parents led to greater feelings of closeness with his siblings for the years their children were growing up, but because they lived in different cities and had different interests, their ties remained tenuous.

Mr. W liked the people his siblings had married and he felt that they genuinely liked his wife. Occasionally, the entire clan would vacation at the patient's enclave in Maine, and Mr. W remembered these times with great pleasure and pride, almost as if he had assumed his father's role as head of the family. But the visits were few and infrequent, and the siblings drifted apart, much to the patient's consternation. At any rate, he thought, he had his own family, and they were a great pleasure to him. He delighted in the way his wife would hug and kiss the children, although in their lovemaking, he maintained the physical reserve he had grown up with. His problem with physical closeness often was onerous, he felt, but he was unable to modify this in his relationship with his wife. He acknowledged later that he had never considered the idea that she might be unhappy about his difficulties with intimacy; it was more a matter of his own inability to overcome a problem of concern to him.

As the years went by, Mr. W and his flying buddy G rose in their company. His friend ultimately became chairman, and the patient became senior executive and manager of the firm's most important division. Things went smoothly for the company for many years, until a series of unexpected setbacks occurred. Increases in world oil prices and concomitant disturbances in relations with nations who were important suppliers of raw materials for the company led to acute shortages and difficulties in producing and marketing the company's major products. The patient, his friend, and the other directors of the company did what they could, but the company eventually went bankrupt. It was a bitter time for the patient and he found himself withdrawing more and more into his shell.

When the patient's coronary occurred, this withdrawal deepened rapidly. His problem with physical intimacy also seemed to worsen, and he sensed that he was shutting his wife out, but he was unable to do anything about it. Dreams of his heart attack left him feeling as if he were sitting on the edge of his life, ready to fall into some bottomless precipice. When the first inklings of the bankruptcy arose, V had tried to reach out to her husband to help and to talk, but he had been unable to respond. His wit and verbal ability seemed to have disappeared and he felt drained and silent. By the time he had his heart attack, his wife's gestures seemed merely perfunctory. In spite of his awareness of their worsening relationship, Mr. W was genuinely shocked when his wife told him that she was leaving him. Some time after this, he was referred to me.

When I first saw Mr. W, he stared intently at me for a moment and started to stretch his arm out, as if to shake my hand, but then seemed to think better of it. A moderately large man and somewhat overweight, he was nearly 6 feet tall and weighed about 190 pounds. His face was pale and his eyes and hair were deep brown. He had an interesting face, especially when an occasional smile lit his eyes. His features were regular and substantial, suggesting a reservoir of strength beneath his impassive exterior.

Mr. W's voice seemed halting and uncertain at first, as if he had not spoken aloud for a long time. He was also ambivalent about opening himself up to a "stranger." "I'm not used to this sort of thing," he noted. "If my whole world hadn't come tumbling down around me now, it's unlikely that I'd be here." He then spoke of the loss of his wife, his job, his health, and the solidity of his world. "Can you get them back for me, doctor?" he asked. And his eyes misted over until he straightened up and cleared his throat.

With very little prodding, he offered most of the details I have recounted. Amidst his successes and his failures, the thread of his problem with physical intimacy, or more aptly, with physicality per se, stood out like a red flag.

"I feel like an old plane in need of hangar time. In my lifetime, I've mostly waited for circumstances to dictate the choices I've made. I'd like to change that now, only I'm not sure how to do that, or if I can.

"After the business folded, and I had my heart attack, I felt as if I were waiting for the inevitable to happen with my wife, and I wasn't doing anything to prevent it. I think I expected the squadron to fly in and save me, the way the war did with my job at the bank. I can't really blame V for leaving me, though I clearly resent the way she did it. Can you make me over, doc? Can you put a new prop on the old mind and body?"

When I first began to see the patient, I was in my late forties, about 15 years younger than he was. Although I prided myself on being in relatively good physical condition, I, too, was aware of some "wear and tear" on the "old machine," which made me more empathetic to him than I might have been, had I been ten years younger.

In addition, I too, had learned to fly in the service, and planes and all their lore and mystique had long been important to me. As small children, my only brother (who was older) and I had flown with a pilot friend of my father's in open cockpit biplanes from World War I. The memories of those first flights still lingered. I had also crash-landed a plane on one occasion, which enhanced my empathy to the patient. More importantly, though, my brother (also a World War II veteran) was slowly dying at the time I first began to see Mr. W, and the rescue fantasy that had been so important in my countertransference feelings with Mr. T was re-activated in my early reactions to Mr. W.

The patient's homely image of asking me to give him a new prop for his old mind and body appealed to me and to my sensibilities. His obvious wish, for me to replenish his life and his masculinity with my therapeutic phallus, predisposed me to think of his problems as stemming from the oedipal phase of development, rather than from a more primitive level. I realized that this might not be the case, but something in the imagery and in my wishes to rescue my dying brother and to resurrect my dead father helped me to so interpret his statement and to play down the significance of some of his more negative signals. Yet it was hard to disregard these signals for long, for they spoke volumes about the depths to which the patient's self-esteem had fallen. One example of such a signal came when Mr. W said:

"I've been wounded badly by life, doc, in more ways than I can count. I've got oak leaf clusters on my oak leaf clusters on my purple heart. It'll take more than a new paint job to re-color my view of myself. I don't envy you your task. You've got a hard job in front of you."

The patient's prose was colorful, but it also indicated a rocklike passivity and suggested that he saw me as the one who was to be giving something to him (therapeutic phallus-prop or whatever) and not that we might be partners in the treatment. Although

Mr. W clearly recognized his passivity, and registered his disgust with it, there was little evidence that he felt it could be changed. Even the World War II vintage verbal imagery I found so enticing bespoke of an element of rigidity and of a tug toward the past, not the future. These were not the most encouraging signs in a man of 62, but neither would they be the most encouraging signs in a man of 32.

Yet in my sessions with the man, I was impressed with the ease with which he spoke. He required few, if any, interventions, which belied his apparent passivity. And despite having lost his job, his wife, and some aspect of his health, he had not surrendered totally to his fate. He was still fighting, albeit, quietly. All of this is to say that I was undecided as to what modality of treatment to offer him, psychoanalysis or psychoanalytic psychotherapy. The question was not a difference in their aims, but rather of which one I thought would help Mr. W break through his passivity.

One day I inquired as to whether he recalled any recent dreams. He responded: "I wondered when you'd get around to asking me about that. I've always heard that dreams were one of the prime interests of you fellows. I've had a couple, but I remember only one recently, that I had over the weekend.

"I was with my wife in a plane, a 747 I think. We were sipping drinks and quietly talking and the stewardess was coming down the aisle bringing the trays with dinner for the passengers. Suddenly some men appeared with guns. They looked like PLO types, you know, towel heads. They shoved right past the stewardess and came down the aisle to where V and I were seated and pointed the guns at our heads. Then one of them said something in a language I wasn't sure I understood and he looked over at me rather ominously. I could feel the sweat streaming down my chest and then I woke up."

In his associations, Mr. W immediately related his sweating in the dream to his symptoms during his coronary. "It's different than the other dreams I used to have about the heart attack, the pain and the terror about my heart seem to be blocked out quite a bit in this one. Maybe that's got to do with our talking about all of this in here. I don't know why the hijacking or the PLO types. I must have read about a skyjack in the newspaper recently, or seen one reported on TV. It was nice, though, to be sitting next to V, really comforting. I guess I really would like you to get her back for me."

I asked a number of questions about the PLO men and the stewardess, to see if they reminded him of anyone, but they didn't. My other queries about the details of the dream drew similar blanks. Finally, I commented that there seemed to be two conflicting feelings in the dream, one of comfort, associated with his wife, and one of anxiety, associated with the PLO types. I suggested that perhaps these antithetical trends might have been aroused in his sessions with me and that they might relate to his feelings about what he expected the treatment, with its new and frightening language, to bring.

"You know, doctor," he answered, "I think you have a point there. I like talking to you, but it does scare me. I'm not sure what's going to come up in here. It's a little like going into a power dive and letting someone else hold onto the stick. But I guess I don't have any other choices, do I now?"

Once more the airplane imagery permeated the session, replete with the flagrant phallic pleading that seemed so much a part of the man. He was trusting, all right, to the point of passivity. Would he trust himself right into a corner and thus smother the treatment? I mused over this question and then decided to confront the patient with the nature of his verbal imagery.

"I wonder if you're aware of how often you use imagery about airplanes in your speech?" I asked.

"I've been told that before," he responded, and became silent. "V used to comment on that a lot after my heart attack. She said I was beginning to sound like a broken record of one of my old squadron get-togethers. That was kind of a bitchy thing to say, don't you think?"

"Evidently you felt it was. Did you feel that my question was bitchy, too?"

"No, you had to ask yours. She didn't. You just want me to focus on why I keep on talking about the past, or maybe even living in it. I must sound like the guys who say that their college years were the high points of their lives. I was never that kind of person. I always felt that the best time of my life was the time I was living at the moment. Not the past or the future, but the present. Only I haven't felt that way since everything started to go bad for me. I think I have turned back to the past and away from the present. I don't like that trait in other people. It doesn't sit too well on me, either."

"Of all of the times in the past that you might have chosen to go back to, why the second world war?"

"It was the high point, in a sense. I was a hero. I wasn't an ace or a headline jockey, but I was damn good. V loved me then and my parents did, too, I even felt pretty good about myself."

I was impressed with the swiftness and the directness of the patient's response. He was clearly not that frightened about looking at himself. The availability of the dream also showed that unconscious material was accessible to him and that he could work with it. In addition, from his response to my comments about the dream, he was obviously willing to recognize transference feelings, which spoke well for the possibility of an analytic process. Thus I decided to suggest analysis to the patient.

In this, I was swayed by a number of factors, some of which I have just described. Another factor could best be described as emotional. Here, I would group the rescue fantasies toward my brother and father and the empathic counteridentificatory response I had to the patient's being a pilot. In addition, Mr. W's comment that he guessed that he had no other choices but to trust me struck me as important: He had to be there with me in treatment, he had no other place to go. It was not said with the desperation of a suicidally depressive patient, but rather with quiet conviction about the correctness of the decision—a conviction about the treatment that represented a motivation that I was certain this patient had never had before. As he had said, if his world had not come tumbling down, he would not have been there. It is just this intensity of motivation, that one so often sees in the older patient entering treatment. In a sense, the clock has nearly run out, it is the last chance to get help.

Obviously, Mr. W had a number of strikes against him. He had had a coronary, and one could seriously question the wisdom of embarking upon a course of deeply probing treatment that might lead to both psychological and physical consequences that could shoot out of control and end disastrously. But this could happen in a patient who had never had a coronary, and his internist had pronounced him well enough to embark upon an exercise program, as well as therapy. He was then too passive, but he had been active enough to fly one hundred combat missions over Europe and to have managed an important division in a major company for many years, and he had done his job well. His wife had left him, but he had helped push her away from him; his children and friends, however, were still reaching out to him, despite his difficulties in responding. This indicated his capacity for establishing solid object-relationships. All in all, there were at least as many positive factors as negative ones, so it came down to my feeling that analysis was the only modality of treatment that could affect the patient's passivity.

When Mr. W lay down on the couch for the first time, he smiled slightly and commented: "You know, it's funny talking to you like this, without being able to see you. It's a little like talking to a wing man over the radio or to the man in the control tower. Whoops, there I go again with my airplane talk. Anyway, it's a sensation which I haven't had in years. It'll take me a while to get used to it."

I was impressed at how the patient had responded to my earlier confrontation. Certainly it had not made him give up this verbal imagery. But it had made him aware of it, and that was as much as one could expect under the circumstances.

It took Mr. W very little time to adapt to the process of analysis, to the couch, and to not being able to see me. He spoke easily and freely, with few interruptions for the first several sessions, of his daily routine and of the people who currently made up his life. These consisted of a few old friends and business associates, a few people he met at the athletic club, and his sibs and children. He verbalized the desire to meet someone to share his life with, but expressed doubts that he would be able to deal with a woman, if he did meet one. By this he meant he did not know if he could handle the natural sexual consequences of any liaison. The subject depressed him.

"V really hurt me," he said, "when she said that I wasn't ever really interested in her needs. I guess F [the mutual friend his former wife married] is better at gratifying her than I was. Jesus, I hate to think about that. It almost makes me sick when I talk about it."

The patient expressed these thoughts toward the end of the first month of the analysis. It was clear that thoughts of his former wife were never very far from his awareness. Her departure had hurt him deeply and he was still assimilating the blows to his self-esteem.

"I don't know how she could have said that I never paid any attention to her satisfaction. I was always aware of whether or not she'd had an orgasm. She almost always did. I know I'm not a very physical person, but I thought I was a pretty decent lover. Besides, she knew I was scared and hurting, after the company went under and I had the heart attack, why the hell did she have to add to it then? It was so damned unfair of her. If she'd've only given me some more time, I'd've come around."

This session marked the first occasion the patient expressed any pent-up anger against his former wife. As his anger began to emerge, he would occasionally ask if he had the right to feel what he was feeling, or to express those feelings to me. After all, his wife was not present to defend herself. He took my initial silence as disapproval of his comments. But after I suggested to him that perhaps the disapproval might be his own, he was able to proceed with his escalating diatribe against her.

For the next month or two, his sessions were filled with these recriminations, as well as with vituperations directed against the mutual friend she married. They were initially seen as having hurt him deeply. Then he began to depict his former wife and friend as insensitive souls, oblivious of the humiliation and anguish they had caused him at such a low period in his life. Although the patient seemed to be justified in feeling angry at his former wife and friend, the shift seemed worth noting.

"In listening to your comments about V and F," I finally said, "you keep referring back to the idea of their being so insensitive to your pain, so callous to your needs. While I'm not trying to dispute the correctness of those points at all, I wonder if there isn't something else that you're also expressing in your statements about them. Do you have any of those same feelings in here with me?"

Mr. W thought about what I had said and then replied, "Not at all, doctor, you're really exquisitely sensitive to my needs. I'm really glad to have you to listen to me."

The next day, when he came in for his session, he said: "I know you didn't mean it that way yesterday, but I somehow felt as if you were criticizing me for what I'd been saying about V, for being so angry at them. I know you're not asking me to defend myself for being angry. You said so yourself, yesterday, but I still felt that."

I realized that the patient had blocked the transference significance of my comment to him, which surprised me. He had seemed to be so cognizant of transference in his early responses to the dream during the evaluative phase of treatment. I was puzzled as to just how he saw me as being insensitive to his needs now. The issue was clarified a few days later when I noticed him glancing at his watch as he entered.

"Must have been quite a session with that lady," he noted, as he lay down on the couch.

I realized then that I had run over a few minutes with the preceding patient, a female patient in her late 40's. Mr. W was obviously angry about that. I thought back for a moment and realized that I had probably done this on other occasions when I had seen her before him. Obviously, he felt slighted. When I asked him about this, I realized that the question had hit the mark.

"It does bother me when you do that," he said. "I get the feeling that you care more about her than about me. I guess I need to feel that I have all of your attention when it comes to my time. I suppose I mean to say that my time is my time and not hers."

I wondered aloud if the woman who preceded him resembled his former wife. Again, the comment struck home.

"She's not as pretty as V, but the overall feeling is very much the same. It seems a little crazy to me to get all that excited about a couple of minutes time, but I guess I do want to feel that you're on my side and not on hers. Somehow that's important to me."

I decided to watch my time with him more carefully, but I also wondered if there were some particular reason why I had favored the woman who preceded him and slighted him. When I thought about it, I concluded that his passivity had bothered me more than I had realized. Could I really give him what he seemed to need from me? When I thought that over, I realized that I was once more displacing certain feelings of frustration about the course of my brother's illness onto the treatment of Mr. W. The incurable nature of the one problem was making it difficult to handle the other. When I understood the connection, the unconscious slighting of the patient disappeared.

Some weeks later, Mr. W came to his session looking somewhat unkempt. He had not shaven and his shoes were less briskly polished. In addition, he appeared to have larger than usual circles under his eyes.

"I'm tired," he commented. "I slept very poorly last night. My brother's wife called to say that he's been hospitalized because of abdominal pain. They're going to operate tomorrow, but there's a pretty good chance he's got cancer. I'm really upset by the news. Even though we haven't been all that close in recent years, N's a very sweet guy." He began to cry then. "He's a young man. Too young to. . . ."

I had the feeling that this latest situation would add to my problems in handling my countertransference feelings toward him. It was upsetting to see the startling parallels in our lives.

The patient flew to his brother's bedside for a few days. When he returned, he was happy. The surgery had revealed that the brother was suffering from a rather exotic, but benign tumor. His brother had been pleased with his visit and the family reunion was complete when his sister had arrived. It was the first time in a while that all the siblings had been together and the pleasurable resolution of their anxieties drew them closer. This happy ending also allowed me to achieve the necessary distance from the patient and his life situation, to enable me to more thoroughly analyze my own countertransference problems, and to more firmly set them to rest.

"It was really nice being with the two of them," Mr. W commented. "It was the first real sense of family that I've felt for a long time. It reminded me of the summers we used to spend in Maine with all the kids. God, those were good days. There I go again, looking back at the old days. Sis picked up the same thing that you did, the airplane terms. She told me that I ought to turn my gaze toward the future and not look back at the past. She's right, I know, but it's not an easy thing to do."

This visit brought a return of the kinds of sessions in which Mr. W verbalized his anger toward his ex-wife. She had broken a bond, a sacred trust, and the entire fabric of their lives together was suspect. He had imagined her to be a different kind of person, someone to whom loyalty and friendship were enduring virtues. And she was obviously not that kind of person, particularly in view of her adulterous involvement with F, their snakelike friend.

In his polemics against his wife and his former friend were a number of accurate self-appraisals. He had obviously contributed to the demise of the relationship by his withdrawal, he realized, his damned turning inward on himself. And the subtle sexual rejections of V must have really hurt her, although he had not meant it personally. He just could not help himself at the time. How could he perform like a man when he did not see himself as a man? In one sense he didn't blame her, and in another he blamed her with a searing intensity. Would he ever get over the hurt she had inflicted on him, he wondered? He was not certain.

At this phase in the treatment, few references to the transference were available. Dreams were uncommon and were not especially revelatory in content. Mostly we were dealing with a rehash of his bitter rejection at the hands of his ex-wife. Then shortly before I was to go away for a brief spring vacation (the patient had been in analysis for just over six months), Mr. W reported the following dream:

"I was walking on a kind of barren plain. No vegetation was visible at all and the ground was pock-marked, as if a stream of small meteors had struck the place in some ancient time. Black basalt rocks were strewn about, giving the area the appearance of a lunar landscape. I felt cold in the dream, despite the fact that I was dressed warmly in woolen pants, long johns and a fleece-lined jacket.

"It seemed as if I had been walking about for a long time, though I had the sensation that I hadn't really gotten very far. Then my gaze was drawn upward, toward the sky and there was a beautiful light there that attracted me. I stretched my hands up in the direction it was coming from and suddenly I became aware of another presence in the dream, behind me. I think it was you, though I didn't really see you. It drew me back down to the black landscape, away from the light. You must have spoken some words, I guess, though I don't have any recollection of exactly what you said. When I looked up at the sky again, though, the light was gone and it felt very, very cold. I must have awakened myself then, because I was shivering and the covers were on the floor."

The intensity of the imagery surprised me. None of the loneliness and desolation depicted in the dream had been presented in recent sessions. Nor was the dream one of his typical productions, which were largely populated by friends and relatives. Curious as to what the day's residues for the dream might have been, my unspoken question was answered in short order.

"G's dead," Mr. W announced, in a funereal voice. "He had a heart attack while he was playing tennis at the club yesterday. He died in the ambulance. His wife called me to let me know. The funeral is tomorrow, so I'll have to miss my session with you."

G was the patient's former flying buddy and best friend, as well as his former business associate. The two had lived through so much together and the one's death sent a frightful chill through the other. Not even the fleece-lined flight jacket in the dream had proven warm enough to ward off the patient's resurgent fears of his own death, linked as they were to this latest loss.

"I really loved him, you know," the patient said. "In many ways, we were closer than I am to my brother, or to anyone else. I'll miss him so much, it scares me. I think he must have been the light in the dream, or maybe the light is all the things from the past that seemed so bright and beautiful once. And you're the killjoy who breaks the spell and keeps drawing me back down to earth. Only its more like the forgotten moon of some far-off planet. It's as if I've traveled some infinite distance, but I haven't really gotten anywhere at all. Maybe that's what's going on in here with the two of us. I talk and talk and talk, and it seems as if I'm getting somewhere, only I'm really going in circles and I keep coming back to my starting spot."

"Do you think," I asked, "that there might be some connection between the desolate feeling that you're experiencing now, and that you felt in the dream, and the fact that I'll be going away on vacation next week?"

"I can't believe you," he responded angrily. "Atomic bombs could be landing all around us and you'd still be asking if the shock waves were related to some damned move of yours. In case no one's ever told you this before, you really are self-centered as hell."

The patient lay in stony silence throughout the rest of the hour and was out the next day at his friend's funeral. When his silence continued through the early portion of the following session, I inquired about his thoughts.

"I'm not thinking about much," he said, in a sullen voice. "I just want to get these couple of days over with, so I don't have to contend with you for a while."

"To contend with what about me?" I asked.

"Your self-centeredness," he responded. "You know what I'm talking about."

"Is it really so self-centered to imagine that my going away next week might link up with the death of your friend? Or that the blackness of the lunar landscape in the dream might be connected to the black color of my couch? I wonder if it's occurred to you that you may want me to draw you back down to earth in the dream, cold and dark as it may seem to be, as I may seem to be right now, because we still represent a connection to life and not a link to death."

The patient seemed shaken by my interpretation and began to shiver slightly, almost as if he had returned to the milieu of the dream. And then he stopped shivering and the tears began to stream down his cheeks.

"You're right," he said, "it does scare me that you're going away. It's as if there's no one here to protect me from the recurrence of the pains, the possibility of death. I'm frightened. I wish that you wouldn't go. Funny, I think the long johns I was wearing in the dream were really a reference to you. I keep thinking that you're going skiing next week. Are you? Won't you please tell me? I don't want to be all alone right now. I don't want to die."

It felt strange for me to listen to Mr. W then. He was a man in his 60's, yet his pleadings had a quality that made him seem like a little boy. And a frightened little boy, to boot. For the separation from me seemed like a death warrant to him. My awareness of the intensity of his dependency on me startled me. I realized that I was feeling guilty about leaving my brother when I went away. I wanted to deny his helplessness and his dependency, his childish quality. And my denial had carried over to the patient, hence my being startled by my recognition of his dependency on me even after I had just interpreted it to him.

The patient interrupted my reverie. "You know," he said, "I don't think that the black color in the dream only relates to the color of your couch. I think that it has something to do with my mood, as well. I've really felt pretty black, pretty lousy for the past few days, as if I despair of ever finding anything good to brighten up my life again. It makes me angry to think that kind of thought. I don't want everything to be over with. That's why I came to see you, why I began the analysis. Only you haven't really changed anything. You're not any more able to conquer death than I am. I envied you your age when I first started with you. Maybe some of the talk about World War II was to undo the sense of envy toward you. But no matter what the difference in our ages is, you still won't be able to beat death either. So what good are you, really? You might as well go away, it doesn't really matter."

His rapid oscillations in mood continued until I did go on vacation. He alternated between feeling sad at the thought of my impending absence and denying that my going away had any significance. Shortly before the last session prior to my vacation was over, he voiced some further feelings of loss about his friend. He cried unashamedly as he spoke of their long-standing devotion and their mutual support and loyalty. In his praise of his friend, his condemnation for my leaving him was clear. For the time being, I was lumped with his ex-wife, among the legions of the disloyal.

When I returned from my holiday, he received me with disinterest, in the manner of a child punishing a returning parent. He made no mention of my trip for a few sessions and simply detailed some of his activities during my absence. After so treating me for what he deemed a sufficient period of time, he returned to the theme of loss and sadness attendant upon the death of his friend.

"G was the warmest guy I ever knew," Mr. W said, "with the possible exception of his father. They weren't phony backslappers, either. When they touched you, it went right through your skin, to your very innards. Not like my family. With my parents, their kisses glanced right off your cheeks. And their embraces never encircled you and held you tight, as G's and his father's did, they just sort of eased on by you tangentially and managed to usually miss the mark."

Mr. W's graphic description of his friend and of his own family evoked a series of images in me that paralleled the scenes he had been describing. It was somewhat like listening to a dream and envisioning the scenario. I was deeply moved by the intensity of the imagery and I felt more attuned to the patient and to his needs than I had before my vacation.

A couple of weeks later, Mr. W told me that he would be having lunch with a "headhunter" to talk about working for a small consulting firm—a group of individuals from diverse business backgrounds, although most of them had a reasonable degree of expertise in marketing. He seemed excited by the possibility. "After all," he said, "it's the first concrete prospect that's come my way in years."

The lunch and the interview with the group went quite well and an invitation to join them was extended. The work entailed some traveling, which cut into the analytic schedule, but it seemed reasonable for the patient to be away at those times. Being back at work seemed to rejuvenate Mr. W. He appeared quite a different person than the one who had been plaintively bemoaning the loss of his friend a few months before. His energy returned and the passivity that had threatened to engulf him in his years of inactivity was very little in evidence. The transformation was really quite remarkable; he actually looked years younger.

In the analysis, the sessions seemed to center about whatever his current business concerns were. Would he get the business he was pitching at a particular company? Would they like his approach (es)? How would he relate to the different personalities? Despite the seeming anxieties such questions might suggest, he functioned well, and his intelligence and expertise became quite apparent to all.

Unfortunately for the fledgling firm, the national economy was undergoing a serious downturn and many large businesses were caught in a cash flow crisis because of the high cost of borrowing money. This seriously crimped their utilization of outside consultants and led to a necessary retrenchment on the part of the small group Mr. W had joined. With great reluctance, he was let go, even though he had performed well.

Contrary to my expectations, Mr. W was not nearly as shaken by this as I had assumed he would be. He gritted his teeth and made the rounds of "headhunters" leaving his updated resumes, and then checking to see if they had followed through on any of the leads they had spoken to him about. It seemed as if his few months in the field of the gainfully employed had changed his outlook on life remarkably. Then it was time for my summer vacation, and the black mood of the early spring seemed to descend once more. And again, as on the earlier occasion of G's death, the change in his spirits was first manifest by the occurrence of a frightening dream.

"I was in a large office building. . . . A little like one of the business places I'd been to, when I was doing consulting. I opened the door to one of the offices, and when I stepped inside, it was no longer an office building but a hospital. I had walked into an operating room of sorts, and they were performing open heart surgery on a patient. Only somehow it involved his face, too. I couldn't really get a good look at him, but I had an uncanny feeling that the man on the table was me. The surgeons seemed to be chatting together, about one thing or another, seemingly oblivious to the state of the poor wretch on the table. . . . I couldn't stand watching the scene, it scared me too much. But when I tried to turn and go, my feet were rooted to the spot and I was unable to move. Then I woke up in a panic."

In his associations to the dream, Mr. W referred to the fact that the failure of the consulting firm had taken the "heart" out of him. It was so discouraging to be buoyed up one moment and then dragged back down to earth the next. The world really was indifferent. What he had said about V in the past, was just as true for almost everyone else, with the possible exception of G, and he was dead. The doctors in the dream certainly didn't care about the man they were working on.

When he stopped there, I observed that his feelings about the indifferent attitude of doctors must be related to the fact that we would be stopping soon for the summer vacation break. I did not comment that his statement of being dragged back down to earth was likely a recurrence of his preoccupation with flying. It seemed most prudent to concentrate on one thing at a time.

"You're right," he said, "I am angry at your going away. You certainly do have a lousy sense of timing. You're a professional and this is your job, but you don't really care about me as a person. How could you? It'd be too trying to let that many different people into your life, all demanding something, all wanting a piece of you. But if you're not prepared to give some small piece of yourself, dammit, then you shouldn't be in this business in the first place."

The patient continued for some time with his diatribe. I wondered just what piece of me he really wished me to give him. When he finally stopped speaking, I inquired about the part of the dream in which the surgery involved the patient's face as well as his heart.

"Still doing your job," he answered sullenly. "I don't really know what they were doing to his face. It was as if they were stripping thin sheets of skin off of it, almost as if he'd been burned and they were trying to get down to the good healthy tissue which lay below the surface."

"That almost sounds like a description of what we're attempting to do in here," I observed.

"Only I'm the one who's stripping myself bare and you're not. I tell you all about myself and I don't know a damned thing about you. I don't even know where you're going on your summer vacation. It's not very fair."

"Does anything particular that you might want to know about me come to mind?"

"I don't know. Whether you're married, I guess. Do you have any kids of your own? Are you and your wife having any problems?"

"Meaning in bed?"

"Yes."

"In other words," I said, "how similar are our lives and our difficulties."

"Yes, for Christ's sake. Can you really understand me, if your wife thinks that you're the greatest lover that's ever populated God's green earth? If your life's been a series of successes crowning successes, how can you relate to a man a good 15 years older than you are, who's on the downhill side of the curve?"

"And the only answer that you can come up with to that question, is that I do it in a dispassionate and clinical manner. What you seem to want is for me to be as rooted to the spot as you are in the dream, for me not to ever want to leave you. And the only way that you can comprehend that I might be interested in doing that, is for me to be as wounded as you see yourself as being."

This interchange with the patient was certainly the most direct expression of his dependency on me in the analysis thus far. Yet it seemed to accentuate the poignancy of his depression. He seemed listless in his sessions. The anger he had vocalized following the dream was nowhere in evidence in the days and weeks that followed. I was concerned about him when the time came for me to leave. He seemed even more apathetic than he had been when he had commenced the analysis. Although I was not apprehensive about the possibility of suicide, I was not sure that his ego might be too fragile for the rigors of the treatment.

When I returned from my vacation in the fall, Mr. W was essentially unchanged. He seemed tired and appeared slightly unkempt. His eyes did not meet my gaze when he walked into the office and he lay down on the couch with an air of resignation.

"It's been a discouraging month," he said, "even the weather was lousy. Too damned hot. I'm not sure I want to continue with this treatment very much longer. I've learned things, but it's not getting me very far."

The patient's voice was not angry as he spoke. It seemed evenly modulated and reticent. I felt I had to strain a bit to catch all of his words. In a certain sense, Mr. W never ceased to surprise me. So often his moods were at variance with what I expected them to be. Just when I felt that I had a good reading as to where he was, he appeared in a different guise, in a new location. I had an image of being in an aerial dogfight, in which I was trying to locate him in my gunsights, only he was never there long enough for me to take aim. The irritation I was feeling with him in the image was certainly not lost upon me.

I wondered about my irritation. Why was I feeling angry with him? Was I demanding that he get well? Or that I might have more control over his moods? I was uncertain of the answer to my questions, but my irritation seemed to abate with my having asked them of myself.

After a few days in which Mr. W spoke again of leaving the analysis, he decided to remain with it "at least a little bit longer." He still seemed relatively apathetic for a number of weeks, but he began to pay more attention to his dress and his personal appearance. "Even if I don't feel any better," he said, "I can try and look the part."

The idea of trying to look the part, which was a type of thought the patient later associated with his father's outlook on life, ushered in a period of several months in which he spoke a great deal about his parents. It was hard for him to feel truly angry at them. They had never been mean or destructive, rather, they had simply been too WASPy, too cold, too elusive. Everytime he tried to reach out and grasp hold of their images in his mind, they were gone. There were memories of the two of them, or of each individually, which seemed to swim with warmth, but when he tried to sample the water, it turned cold or dried up. He described them one day as a pair of missiles he was tracking, only they had no heating system to hone in upon.

From the patient's description, I realized the origin of my own difficulties in locating him in my "gunsights." I told him of my thoughts, in the sense of informing him of how difficult he, too, was for me to find on the tracking screen. I noted that in his identification with the mechanism utilized by his parents, he was expressing his deep-seated longing for ties to them. I further noted that his own elusiveness must have posed difficulties for his family and friends, which then probably interfered with the warmth and love he might receive from them in return.

He found my comments quite meaningful. He had never really looked on himself as difficult to know. Quite the contrary, he said, he thought of himself as being as easy to read as an open book. You could usually take one glance at him and know what his mood was. It suprised him to know that people such as me might want to know more than what was on the surface, such as what led to the different transfigurations of the surface.

Maybe his ex-wife was not really the bitch he had portrayed her as being. She might actually have had justifiable grievances against him, which she had been unable to express in any other way. But the mutual friend was still a "son of a bitch," no matter which way you cut it, "to do that to a good friend."

In his dreams that fall, Mr. W often visited childhood locales, frequently seeing himself as both a child and as an adult. In the latter representation, he was a dispassionate observer, in the manner of his parents with him then, or of the analyst with him now. After a number of such dreams, he had one in which the patient as observer representation began to move his arms toward the patient as child representation in the dream, but before he could actually touch him, he awoke with feelings of anxiety.

"I don't know why that scared me quite so much," he said, "but I could barely sleep the rest of the night."

"What occurs to you?" I asked.

"It was almost as if you were reaching out, not me," he answered.

"Why was that so frightening?"

"I don't know. On the one hand, it's just what I've been asking you to give to me. The warmth that my parents never managed to get across. On the other hand, there's something about your actually doing it that...."

The patient stopped in mid-thought, more in the manner of someone who was confused as to just what thought would follow, than in the manner of someone who was withholding his thoughts. My own associations had jumped ahead to the homosexual meaning of the gesture to the patient, but he once more guessed the nature of my musings.

"Maybe it's got some kind of homosexual connotation to me," he observed, "the idea of your reaching out and touching me. Only why wouldn't that have come up with G or with his father? I'm confused right now."

Over the next few weeks, he came to accept that his desire to be close to me did have a sexual aura about it, although the thought of actually sleeping with a man was abhorrent. Shocking as it might have seemed to him some time in the past to verbalize this, he could actually imagine being locked in an embrace with another man. A kind of bear hug, wherein the warmth of the one person could be communicated to the other. He had seen Europeans do this, and even American fathers and sons or good friends. G and his father had hugged each other when they greeted each other after a long period of being apart, although they would not hug him. They had intuited his reserve and had only gone as far as putting their arms about his shoulders. Why the hell hadn't his own father been able to be more physical with him, to embrace him, he wondered? he knew he would have been a better person for the experience.

Despite the progress in the patient's capacity to be in touch with his desires for masculine closeness, little seemed to be occurring in the patient's life outside the sessions. He spent Thanksgiving with his son's family and Christmas with his daughter's. They were enjoyable times and he was pleased to be with his children and grandchildren. But the holiday invitations had come to him; he had not sought out any new people or expanded his relationships with old acquaintances.

In a session after the New Year's holiday, Mr. W bemoaned his loneliness. He noted how seldom the telephone rang in his apartment, which was quiet as a tombstone. The bleak image was a metaphor for his passivity, I thought, but perhaps it was more than that. And then I realized something about the patient's fantasies. If he could only stay perfectly motionless and uninvolved, time would stand still for him. And, perhaps, so would death. The opportunity to test my hypothesis came a few days later.

"I had a call from P [a male friend]," the patient said. "He wondered if I'd be interested in going out with his wife's cousin. She is recently widowed. She sounded rather nice, but I told him that I had to think about it."

"What are your thoughts about it?" I asked.

"I can't really get all that excited about going out with anyone. I think that I'd rather just sit at home. When I went out in the past, I couldn't wait for the evenings to end, so that I could get home. Why should I bother putting myself in that situation again?"

I sat in silence as the patient pleaded the case for his passivity. He went on to talk of how bored he was with most new women he met, they didn't really match V in beauty or charm or grace. No matter how angry he was with her, he guessed that he was still hooked on her. The same thing could be said for the new male acquaintances at the athletic club. He could converse with them or even joke a bit, but he found it impossible to feel a real sense of closeness with any of them. Maybe it was still the barriers that we had been talking about so much in recent months, and the sexual connotation that closeness carried with it.

"I have the impression that it's more than that," I said, after he was quiet again. "More than just your fears of homosexuality with men and sexual performance failures with women. I don't mean to minimize the anxieties those thoughts arouse in you, but I believe that there are also other anxieties which are troubling you."

Once more, Mr. W was silent. And then he replied. "If you mean my fears of death, you're right. I have the theory that for me to start again, means to open up my arms to death. This way, I may be in limbo, in some kind of suspended animation, but it's safe. I know this probably sounds crazy to you, but I think it's what I've felt ever since I had the heart attack. It's almost as if you're only allotted so much safe activity in your life and then if you go beyond that, you're tempting fate. It's dangerous. I've had my quota. I was almost glad when the consulting firm ran out of money for me. I'd had the feeling that I'd been pushing my luck in that direction."

Although his statements paralleled my own thoughts to a considerable degree, his idiosyncratic extensions of those thoughts startled me. Once more, he would not allow himself to be fixed even for an instant in the crosshairs of the gunsight. His comments did explain why he had not been upset as I had expected him to be, after he had lost the consulting job. As I digested that thought, I realized that what the patient had just said had an even greater relevance to a more general area he and I had spoken of many times in the past 16 months.

"If I understand what you're saying to me now," I observed, "you're drawing a parallel between being actually engaged in life and the number of missions you can safely fly without getting shot down. It's as if in each sphere of your life, you only get up to a hundred missions to fly. And if you stretch your luck beyond that, you're a dead man. I have to assume that you feel that you've had your hundred missions in combat, in business and with women, so now it's time to just sit still and blend in with the woodwork. Otherwise the sword will fall and you want to avoid that at all costs."

The patient was silent for a long time. "You know," he said finally, "I'm really impressed with what you just said. You really do understand me, maybe better than I understand myself. There's something about the way that you put it that just cuts right through all of the crap and goes to the very core of things. That's a funny word for me to use right now, to the core, the heart. I really am scared of dying."

As we began to expand upon this theme, we came to see that his hundred combat missions in World War II had to represent what had been a long-standing difficulty, his fear of taking chances, of striking out in new directions. To have been a novelist, as he had thought of being for a brief moment in college, would have put him at odds with his father's value system, and he would have felt guilty and alone, as with other choices he had made. He was surprised, in retrospect, that he had actually stood up to his parents about his choice of V and about not going back into banking after the war.

In discussing this topic, I suggested that the patient appeared to equate the notions of being free, and of taking chances, with doing something wrong and with the feeling of guilt. To fly the hundred and first mission was not simply to spit in the face of death, but also was a temptation to fate and a provocation for some dreadful punishment. In my mind, it was both a fantasy of fusion with a mixed maternal–paternal imago, with a consequent loss of individuality and identity (his fear of death) and an illusion of oedipal triumph, wherein he had killed his father and claimed his mother as his own (with the retaliatory fear of death that accompanied the fantasy being concomitant with his intense castration fears). Although I did not mention these latter thoughts to the patient, he readily responded to the notion that his passivity protected him from coming to grips with his underlying sense of guilt.

"I never thought about it in those terms," he said, "until you brought up the idea of feeling guilty, but it just feels so right and I can't deny it. It's an absolutely true idea and it feels that way to my very depths. I've been guilt-ridden all of my life and I've never even realized it. It's incredible!"

As he talked on, he dredged up a variety of incidents throughout his life, in which he did recall small increments of conscious guilt. Most of them were petty failures, as when he had disappointed friends or relatives in some minor way. Occasionally, the episodes were hard to evaluate, as when he claimed that he had failed to fly close enough to a buddy's wing in combat and the man had been shot down by a German plane. The orgy of blame that followed seemed disproportionate to the degree of failure described, particularly since the mission had been flown in foul weather and his Mustang had been dangerously low on fuel. But again, the simple verbalization of the episode eased his conscience. It was as if he had to recite all the crimes he had "committed," in order to expunge them from his soul and feel free again.

The daily recitations were of such importance to Mr. W, that he barely paused long enough, when the time came for my annual spring vacation, to be upset at the thought of my departure. He told me that he would miss me, but he realized that it would only be a week and that I must need the time away from my work. It seemed quite a change to me from the earlier two pre-vacation periods.

Unfortunately, the vacation proved more traumatic for me than for the patient. I took a nasty spill while skiing during a snowstorm, and came back to the office in a rather imposing-looking cast. As I hobbled about from my chair to the door, I drew an interesting variety of comments from my patients, running the gamut from sympathy to anger.

Mr. W took one look at me and said "You cracked up skiing." When I was silent, he continued. "Will you be able to go back to it again?"

I was surprised when I quickly responded yes to his query. I knew that part of this was a need of my own to master the anxieties aroused in me about the accident, as to whether I would be able to ski again. But I knew also that my answer was also something of a reassurance to the patient. I was saying, in essence, that it was all right to take a chance and even to get hurt, because not every wound is necessarily a "mortal" one. The tension in his voice eased after I said yes, but I knew that we would hear a great deal more about the incident.

And hear about it we did. Mr. W spoke of feeling guilty about my accident, as if in some magical way he had "caused" it. He knew that that was ridiculous, but he found it hard to shake the thought. He had been angrier at me than he had let on, before my vacation. Yet he had also meant what he had said, about my needing the time to get away from my patients and my work. I looked tired to him. Although he recognized the unrealistic quality of the guilt that he was feeling, the feeling itself felt familiar. Only he could not quite place when he had experienced it before.

Approximately six weeks after my return from vacation, when the cast was off my leg and I was walking about without any difficulty, the patient came into his session one day complaining of a twisted ankle. He had incurred the injury to his leg while playing squash at the athletic club. He had had it bandaged by someone at the club, but it still hurt him. He asked me for the name of an orthopedic man and in response to my asking about the injury, he asked:

"Do you think this is another example of my needing to punish myself because I felt guilty about your being hurt? Sounds silly, doesn't it? But I really believe that it's true."

That night, after seeing the orthopedist, and having a lightweight cast applied to his ankle to minimize the swelling, he had a dream. In it, he was playing squash with a fellow member of the club and the struggle for each point became so intense, that it seemed a matter of life and death. With each stroke, he reached for the ball to the very limit of his ability, and he was aware of having taken an almost sadistic pleasure when he heard the sound of the ball cannonading off the back wall toward his opponent. The contest reached such dramatic proportions that he knew that one of them must soon drop from exhaustion or death. Then suddenly it was at match point, and as the ball came rocketing back toward him, he gathered every ounce of strength in his body to make the superhuman lunge for it, which he did. He felt the pain course through his body in the dream, from his ankle to his heart and he awoke in terror.

"That was as scary a dream as I've had in years," Mr. W announced, after he finished describing it. He was quiet for a moment, and then he continued. "It's hard for me to believe that I have such incredibly strong urges to kill you. The anger and the competitive strivings in that dream are the strongest I've ever felt in my life. Not even combat came close to eliciting that much intensity from me."

"I was the man you were playing squash with?" I asked, as a point of clarification.

"Yes. Or if it wasn't you, it was a younger man at the club who reminds me a lot of you in the way that he looks and talks. I can still hear the sound of the ball, rifling off of the wall. It was like a gun exploding. You don't really hear very much in aerial combat, but you can feel it when you're firing your machine guns. Your whole body fires them, not just your fingers. But that's not really true, what I just said. That's the way it's supposed to feel and be. With me, it was more of that observer sensation that we've spoken about before. God, I must feel so guilty about being aggressive, being angry. I can't believe how guilty I must feel. I don't know whether that was the heart attack or my ankle, or whether I lived or died in the dream, or whether you did either. Whatever happened, it certainly scared the hell out of me."

I commented that part of his hurting himself had to do with his desire to hang onto me. In other words, in his identification with the threatened lost love object (me), he was able to become me (as well as dispose of me) and thus mitigate the sense of loss and atone for the feelings of guilt. I noted that we had spoken of this in the past and I asked if he had any further thoughts about this.

"It's funny that you ask that," he commented. "The other man in the dream, I said that he was either you or someone from the club. Well the man he resembles at the club has the same first name as my father. As a matter of fact, he works for the same bank that my father did. There's got to be something in that. It feels as if I must have wanted to kill my father at some time or other in my life. I feel a little incredulous when I say that because he was hardly an evil man who deserved to die, or anything like that. Then again, neither are you. I can't imagine what he could have done to me, or you either, that would have generated such a response in me."

Nothing more was forthcoming then and the pace of the analysis seemed to slow, as the patient's ankle swelling diminished. Then one day, in late May, Mr. W announced that his friend P had asked him again if he wished to go out with his wife's recently widowed cousin. He told me that he had finally acquiesced and that he would be seeing the woman the following evening. I wondered how the date with the pretty widow would go, following our conversation of killing the oedipal father and analyst so closely.

When Mr. W came into the session after the evening in question, he was smiling. "I had a nice time last night," he announced. "E's really a very nice person."

He described the events of the evening, in which the two of them had gone to dinner in a lovely restaurant and then had gone back to her place for a nightcap. She had told him that she found the whole business of dating very difficult. It was hard for her, after having been married for over 30 years (she ws 57), to fill someone new in on the facts of her life. She also openly admitted to him that the idea of sleeping with someone new made her apprehensive.

Her frankness about her anxieties was refreshing to the patient. He felt that it took some of the edge off his concerns about being able to perform sexually for her. He also acknowledged that he found her a very attractive woman. She was tall and slim and obviously kept her body in good shape. And just in case I was wondering, he was going to see her again over the weekend. They had made plans for dinner and the theatre.

When Mr. W appeared for his session the following Monday morning, he was positively beaming. "We slept together," he announced proudly, "and it went like a dream. I'm really smitten with her."

I found it hard to believe that things had proceeded so fast. I was pleased with the results of the liaison, but once more I thought of the gunsight image and of the elusive missiles being tracked by radar. I was truly beginning to understand how the patient had been able to survive his hundred combat missions over Hitler's Europe.

As he began to describe E in the days and weeks that followed, she seemed like a warm, genuine person. She had three grown children, two of whom lived in New York City and who were happy to see her dating someone as eligible as the patient. Mr. W began to invite friends out for dinner and to introduce his new companion to them and she drew hearty votes of approval from all concerned.

Mr. W's evenings and weekends began to take on the appearance of the busy social calendar one might associate with a man of his age and social background. He and E went off on numerous weekend trips and they planned a long sojourn through Europe in the summer break from the analysis.

Although I was certain that the inception of the patient's liaison with E, in some part, represented an acting out of the anxieties aroused by the oedipal transference relationship with me, there seemed no readily available opportunities in the material he presented to me in sessions in which to interpret this idea to him. I also recognized that I was somewhat loathe to upset the applecart, so to speak, as he seemed to have found a genuinely satisfying and gratifying relationship with E, one I did not particularly care to see devalued. I realized, however, that if it had a solid basis, the love affair with the woman would most certainly withstand the onslaughts of the transference interpretations. Thus it became a question of just where and when to find the opportunity to interpret the transference displacement.

The proper moment did not present itself until shortly before the summer vacation break. The patient was discussing his plans for the European trip he was to take with E. Then he rather casually said: "I had the funniest fantasy last night. I imagined that we'd run into you and your wife in Italy, in Verona, I think. Don't ask me why Verona, of all places. It doesn't ring any bells at all. We all found ourselves staying at the same hotel, The Park, I guess, and we were all going to the opera or a play that evening. Anyway, I introduced you to E and you introduced me to your wife. Then we had a drink at a little restaurant and it was very, very warm and nice."

When I asked if he had any thoughts about the fantasy, he replied: "Nothing much, I guess, except I would like you to meet E sometime. I think you'd like her. I also have the feeling that I owe my being with her to you anyway. We are going to Verona, by the way," he added with a chuckle, "in case you and your wife do come by there this summer."

"Have you been thinking about that?" I asked. "Where we'll be this summer?"

"I recognize the refrain," Mr. W replied, "even though it's been a long time since I last heard the music. Seriously though, no, in response to your question. I haven't given it much thought this year, about where you'll be during the summertime."

"Do you have any thoughts about what opera or play you might have been going to see in the daydream?"

"No, I don't. I did go to Verona once with V a long time ago. We did see something in the Roman amphitheater there, but I don't recall what it was."

"Does Verona itself bring anything to mind?"

"Not to mine, but it obviously does to yours."

"It is rather renowned as the city of Romeo and Juliet, and they often do Shakespeare's plays in the amphitheater there in the summer. *Romeo and Juliet* does clearly deal with the issue of the dire consequences resulting from a love affair that proceeds without the benefit of parental blessing. And in the fantasy, and even now, you state that you would like me to meet E, presumably in part to confer my parental approval. I wonder if we're not dealing with a recrudescence of the feeling that you're doing something wrong and are risking punishment for it. If you can get my approval, then presumably the guilt and anxiety can be lessened."

"But there's nothing that I feel guilty about now!" Mr. W protested, but there was no real vehemence in his voice. Rather it was plaintive, as if he anticipated my discovering some dread secret that would interfere with his relationship with E. When I did not respond, he added: "I love her. Please don't upset things with her. I can't stand the thought of losing another person who means so much to me."

In the last few sessions until the vacation break, Mr. W seemed to be coasting through the hours, as if he were simply treading water. I commented on this to him and he readily acknowledged the point. "I don't want to upset things with E," he said in reply.

"She's just too important to me. I'm sure that you can make a very convincing case for my whole relationship with her being erected as an avoidance of my feelings about you. Maybe that was true in the beginning, but what I feel for her now is real. Let us have the summer together and we'll see what happens when I get back here in the fall."

When he did return in the fall, he spoke glowingly of their summer together. The first session or two sounded like a travelog of a trip through the elegant highways and byways of Europe. Then he returned to the issue of the acting out of the transference.

"I thought a few times during the past month about what we spoke of before I left," he said. "I think you're right. That dream about wanting to kill you or my father in the squash game really scared me. I don't think I realized how much it did at the time. When I considered it, I realized that you could make a very convincing case for my having killed the two of you off so that I could be with E as my mother. Except E's not like my mother at all. She's a warm, loving woman. But her husband's having died fits right into the picture, doesn't it? Maybe that's what its always been about. Maybe that's why I've felt so guilty all of my life. I suppose that outliving all those other guys in combat is pretty much the same thing. But you can only fly so high so often, before you come crashing down. You tuned me into that concept. Remember? Only I'm not quite sure who or what is trying to shoot me down now. Whether it's something inside of me claiming vengeance for my "sins," or you, for reasons which I don't quite comprehend."

"What reasons do you think of?" I inquired.

"I really don't know. I don't really picture you as the jealous type, but I can't really imagine any other explanation. Though Christ only knows what you'd be jealous of. I'm the one who's really jealous of you, your age, your work, the sense of continuity in your life. That's what I want to get back to the most, the sense of meaning and continuity in my life. And the only way that I can really do that is to be in a relationship with a woman whom I love and who loves me and maybe hopefully to find some sort of occupation that would give me a modicum of satisfaction and self-esteem."

Once more, I was struck by the depth of the patient's understanding of exactly what had transpired in the analysis. He had clearly recognized the oedipal motif and keenly understood the acting out of the transference in the inception of his relationship with E. At the same time, however, in so doing this, he had erected a rather rock-ribbed defense against the rigors of treatment. If he stuck to this, I was uncertain as to just how much further we would actually get in the analysis in the foreseeable future.

Time increasingly seemed to prove my prediction. The closer the patient drew to E, the more he defended himself against recognizing any references to the transference. His dreams seemed to be crowded with superficial situations and current characters, and his associations never seemed to deepen our understanding of the present or the past, as they had so often done before. When he made plans to marry at Christmas, I directly asked him if he thought that this might have any effect on the analysis, and he said that he thought it would not. After the honeymoon, however, he suggested that we might consider setting a termination date. I had wondered when this would come up, but there seemed little that could be done about it.

We set a termination date for late spring, a few weeks after my return from my spring holiday. During this period, Mr. W became involved with another consulting group, albeit on a part-time basis. He was pleased to be working again, and the occasional travel his job called for cut still further into his time for analysis. When I pointed this out to him, he expressed his regrets, but felt that it could not be avoided. He did have one further dream of note, however, before we stopped the treatment late in the third year of the analysis.

"I was down in Washington with E. We were strolling through the gardens in Dumbarton Oaks and the cherry blossoms were in bloom. It was very beautiful there, very peaceful. Suddenly I saw G walking toward us and I felt scared for a moment, as if it were a portent of something bad or evil that was going to happen to us. But then he beamed one of those big, broad smiles of his at us and I felt very happy. He shook my hand and kissed and embraced the two of us and his kisses weren't the kiss of death that I had expected, but were infused with warmth and life. It was a really nice dream. I felt happy when I awoke from it."

As I listened to the dream, I realized that Mr. W was expressing his last direct transference wishes toward me in it. I was clearly G in the dream, risen Lazarus-like from the dead to show the patient that separation (from me and from the analysis) was not dangerous.

In addition, I was not really angry at him for leaving me, in the wake of his oedipal triumph with E. On the contrary, I was offering my blessing and my everlasting warmth to the two of them. With practically no prompting from me (in the form of questions about the dream), the patient arrived at most of these same conclusions. He even added that the charter for the International Monetary Fund had been established at a conference at Dumbarton Oaks and that the fund was set up to help alleviate (monetary) problems in member nations. I had helped him to alleviate his problems, but now we were co-equal, member nations, as evidenced by our standing face to face in the dream. When we shook hands at the end of the last session, he grasped my hand in both of his and held it there for a long time.

"Thanks," he said, "You've helped me more than I can ever let you know."

In attempting to list some of the outstanding features of Mr. W's analysis, its abbreviated term stands at the head of the list. Clearly, he left treatment before it could be considered finished. His departure could be seen as a classic acting out of the transference, a cure by love, via the marriage to E.

Yet the marriage seemed a good one, as had Ms. B's relationship with her lover. Both patients were clearly fearful of exploring the intensity of their feelings toward me in the analysis. They both had a greater than average difficulty in handling separations and vacations. Their rage and the attendant guilt feelings were exceptionally painful to both of them. But they both had made enormous headway in their years in analysis.

It would be hard to look at Mr. W's treatment without recognizing the progress he had made. He was able to recognize his lifelong problems with warmth and guilt and to modify both of them significantly. He had gained considerable understanding of his oedipal and pre-oedipal longings and had lessened his fears of castration and of the loss of his sense of individuality. Mr. W was a happier person at the end of the treatment than he had been at the beginning. His marital relationship and job accomplishments seemed quite outstanding, at a time in life when things that good are not all that easy to achieve. Although his passivity was still a major issue, as evidenced by his need to flee treatment, he seemed less concretized in this characterological position and more malleable vis-à-vis the act of actually engaging in life.

6

THE DISSOLUTION OF A FIFTY-YEAR-OLD SYMPTOM: Mrs. R

Mrs. R entered treatment with me at the age of 71, following the death of her former therapist (a man she had spent the prior two decades with, whose psychoanalytic reputation I greatly respected). She expressed mild to moderate feelings of depression, which seemed consistent with the loss of the analyst she had so esteemed. Insomnia, anorexia, weight loss, and suicidal ideas were not present. She also tentatively reported some irritation with her dead therapist for his having abandoned her at this late stage of her life without having cured her of the symptom that had brought her into treatment with him. The symptom referred to was a lifelong feeling, of near delusional intensity, that her son (a man in his late 40's) had been fathered by a black man.

The patient was the eldest of three children born to a Jewish immigrant family living on the lower east side of New York City. Her two brothers were three and five years younger than she was, respectively. Her mother, perceived as a cold, ungiving woman, was seldom home because she worked long hours. Irrespective of her job, however, the mother was always seen as favoring the two male siblings over the patient, although neither brother received an overabundance of maternal largesse. To this day, they both regard the patient as being the most nurturing figure in their early lives.

She considered herself to be her father's favorite until she reached adolescence. At that time, he became crudely vitriolic in his condemnation of any presumed expressions of interest she might exhibit in members of the opposite sex. In juxtaposition to the denunciations of the patient's emerging sexuality was the rather flagrant exhibition of the parents' own sexual interactions. Since the small apartment in which the family lived was crowded, both visual and aural exposures to the primal scene were recalled by the patient, though she was uncertain as to just how young she was when she began to see and hear her parents having intercourse. Definite recollections of such exposures, however, dated back at least to age 10.

As a teenager, Mrs. R began to work as a saleslady in various stores. In one such job, in a clothing store, she spent her salary on clothes for her mother, in the hope of winning the mother's approval. Instead of the approbation she so desperately craved, she was berated by the mother for having squandered her wages, which could have been put to better use to educate her younger brothers.

In her late adolescence, Mrs. R became acquainted with a young black man who cleaned up in one of the stores in which she worked. She liked his ribald sense of humor, and in retrospect, she realized that she had felt distinct sexual stirrings toward him. When she entered her early 20's, she met and became engaged to a poor young Jewish man, whom her parents objected to on the grounds that he lacked initiative. Despite the obvious validity of their objections, and with the knowledge of her suitor's slavish dependency on his tyranical mother, Mrs. R married him when she was 21.

At 23, the patient became pregnant. Her sexual life with her husband left much to be desired and she had never experienced orgasm with him. Sometime during the early part of the pregnancy (which was to be her only one), she either dreamt or had a masturbatory fantasy (we were never able to establish with any degree of certainty just which had occurred) that she had had intercourse with a black man and that this man was the real father of the child she was carrying. At various times (especially when she would become depressed) over the next five decades, Mrs. R would become preoccupied with the idea that an unknown black man had fathered her son. She repeatedly averred, however, that she had always a modicum of reality-testing with regard to this notion and recognized it to be untrue.

The "black man" fantasy depressed her. It also posed a major lifelong stumbling block for Mrs. R in her efforts to love or be affectionate toward her son, toward whom she felt a distinct aversion. At the time that she entered therapy with me, they had a distant, loveless relationship, punctuated with occasional phone calls (he lived halfway across the country) and rare, but unsatisfactory visits by the patient to her son, daughter-in-law, and grandchildren.

Mrs. R had begun seeing her prior therapist because of feelings of dissatisfaction in her life shortly before the death of both her husband and her mother in the same year (when Mrs. R was 50). Although she had expressed the ideas about the black man having fathered her son to her former analyst, he evidently decided against exploring this material psychodynamically. He treated Mrs. R with electroconvulsive therapy when she became depressed after her husband and mother died (although it did not appear, in retrospect, that her symptoms merited this kind of treatment) and with chemotherapeutic agents for her depression when her father died, several years before she began treatment with me. Again at the time of the father's death, she did not show any profound vegetative signs of depression and the tricyclic antidepressive agents she received were never given to her in therapeutically adequate dosages.

Mostly, her treatment with the former therapist consisted of a supportive type of arrangement, with no attempt made to explore either the psychopathological or the transference manifestations she so obviously exhibited. Since the former therapist was dead, and since his notes did not really indicate the reasoning involved in his therapeutic choices, it was not possible for us to understand his rationale for so dealing with Mrs. R's problems. My hunch, however, was that he was following Freud's dictum of not exploring the psyche of a patient over the age of 50 in a psychoanalytic mode.

From the beginning of her treatment with me, the most prominent feature of Mrs. R's therapy was the ready accessibility to consciousness of psychodynamically charged material. All the material presented thus far, in addition to a great deal more, emerged in the first few weeks of this twice-weekly, psychoanalytically oriented psychotherapy. My dealing with the patient was simple. Since the material she was bringing forth did not appear to have any disorganizing or depressing effect upon her, I allowed her to verbalize whatever came to her mind (free association). Although I was surprised by the very early (first two weeks of treatment) appearance of what turned out to be a rather tenacious erotized transference, I believe that my anxiety about this was based more on my own countertransference feelings than on any real need for concern. The idea of Mrs. R's being a woman approximately the age of either my own mother or my own former analyst caused me some difficulty, vis-à-vis the issue of countertransference feelings.

In the third session of the therapy, Mrs. R expounded at some length about her feelings of warmth and love for her prior therapist. She told me how ashamed she had been to reveal to her brothers just how dependent she had become upon him. For example, she had lied to them about her still continuing the treatment with him. She then told me how guilty she had felt at having chosen to visit the former doctor for her regularly scheduled session on the day her husband had passed away in the hospital. This feeling of having erred in her choice arose after the first visit to me, and she had paid a visit to her husband's grave for the first time in many years. Following this visit, she felt somewhat less angry with her husband for having died and with her in-laws, whom she had always despised. This visit marked the beginning of a long overdue process of mourning for these formerly hated objects.

She proceeded to contrast her feelings for her former therapist with her feelings for me. I was characterized at that time as cold, an automaton who absorbed whatever she said without giving back much in return. This was verbalized to me in rather challenging tones, as if I were being dared to exhibit the same degree of warmth toward her her prior therapist had.

"Besides," she added, "you're married. I can see the wedding band on your finger. Dr. X [her former therapist] didn't wear one, so I never knew whether he was or wasn't until after he died and his wife called to cancel our sessions. You . . . you're already spoken for. Nothing could ever happen between you and me."

Because of my reluctance to become directly involved with erotized transference material at this early stage of the treatment, I merely commented about Mrs. R's feelings of loss concerning Dr. X and I wondered if these had been intensified by her having found out that he had been married. She cried briefly in response to my comment and then told me how Dr. X had interfered with her plans to marry a man whom she had met five years before and with whom she had had a deep emotional tie. Sexually, the two of them had enjoyed little pleasure because the man was impotent following a prostatectomy. When he had proposed marriage to the patient, however, Mrs. R felt that Dr. X had insisted that she choose between marrying the man and continuing therapy. Whether this was accurate or not could never be clarified, but the patient never wavered in her rendition of this story. What seems more important to mention, at this juncture, is the fact that the patently obvious paternal transference material that permeated the treatment with Dr. X was never discussed in the therapy sessions.

To return to the session with Mrs. R I was describing: As she reported the unenviable choice apparently posed to her by Dr. X, she spontaneously noted the similarity to her father's vituperative injunctions against sex with boys during her adolescence. It was in this context that she recalled the young black man (and her feelings of sexual attraction to him) who had cleaned up in the store she had worked in some five and one-half decades earlier. Her final comment of the session was to note that her son had been born with a deviated septum, which gave his nostrils a widened, swollen appearance. This was one of the conscious contributing factors in her initial formation of the idea of his having been fathered by a black man. Although all this may sound like a veritable deluge of material to emerge so early in the treatment, at no time was there any sense of pressure or any accompanying feelings of depression or decompensation observable in the patient. She was simply free associating, much in the manner of a younger psychoanalytic patient on the couch.

Over the next few sessions, data relevant to childhood sexual experiences emerged, as when the patient played doctor with a little boy in a nearby apartment. She experienced an upsurge of guilt feelings when she remembered his calling her the Yiddish word for whore, as her father later did during her adolescence. Again, however, this material arose in juxtaposition with memories of sexual arousal with the black man at work and with recollections of both the primal scenes between the parents and a memory of an uncle ejaculating on her buttocks when she briefly shared a bed with him in pre-adolescence. It quickly became apparent to me that the black man theme was obviously related to oedipal incestuous feelings toward her father.

As I debated as to just what to interpret to Mrs. R about the oedipal material emerging in these early sessions, she began to complain of diarrhea during which she became fearful of soiling her undergarments. She developed a transient phobia of riding on the subway to my office (though she never actually avoided this), as she feared not having accessibility to a toilet and perhaps having an "accident." She feared that this would lead to her being shunned by other people for being "dirty" or "smelly." When I inquired as to whether or not she had ever experienced such attacks in the past, she recalled having had severe diarrhea as a child of 10 or 12. As the diarrhea had specifically arisen directly after the session in which the material about the uncle's having ejaculated on her buttocks had emerged, I wondered aloud to her if there might be any connection between these two phenomena. She became embarrassed and then spoke of soiling the sheets with "black feces" while giving birth to her son. I asked if she had ever thought that babies might be delivered per rectum and she answered without hesitation that she had indeed thought so as a child. Concomitant childhood theories of oral impregnation following the swallowing of a "man's seed" were also verbalized.

As the session continued, Mrs. R recalled that on more than one occasion she had seen her father mounting her mother from behind, "like a dog or a monkey," and she further recalled masturbating during early adolescence when looking at some pornographic pictures her father kept in a drawer, in which intercourse was illustrated with the man penetrating the woman from behind. The references to feces and to monkeys led us back once more to the black man theme, but it was becoming more and more obvious to both of us as to just who the indeterminate black man really was. My somewhat circuitous excursion through the genetic determinants of Mrs. R's transference feelings toward me was obviously based on my need to dilute the intensity of the erotized feelings she was expressing to me, because of the multiplicity of responses those feelings aroused in me. Not the least of these was the re-arousal of my own oedipal wishes and the feelings of guilt attendant upon those desires.

The solution to my indecisiveness as to what to interpret to the patient was, as is so often the case, provided by a more direct flowering of the transference itself. Mrs. R became more and more seductive with me during our sessions. She obviously went to a great deal of trouble in choosing her clothing, jewelry, and perfume, and she began to speak of fearing that her talk about her sexual feelings about me might repel me.

When I finally did comment to her that I thought that she might possibly be hoping that I would become aroused by her talk, she became embarrassed, but was able to acknowledge the validity of what I had said. She verbalized the fear that my wife would be angry with her for her attempt to entice me sexually and, in this setting, experienced the urge to defecate and had to leave the office briefly to go to the bathroom.

Upon her return to the office proper, I commented to her that I thought that she must have experienced similar feelings of sexual desire toward her father in the past and must have also feared her mother's wrath, as she now feared my wife's. I suggested that her sexual desires for her father as a child and adolescent may very well have "scared the shit out of her" (the diarrheal attacks of her childhood), especially when she probably wished to take the place of the mother in the primal scenes she had seen in childhood and adolescence, and to have his baby.

These interpretations seemed rather obvious to me, but I was hesitant to make them to the patient. Since we were only in the early weeks of treatment, such deep oedipal interventions felt premature. Although they were accurate, I later realized that the primary reason for my making these comments to her was my need to dilute the current intensity of the erotized transference.

Although I rationalized my reasons for being concerned about the intensity of the rapidly developing transference relationship, I believe that the re-arousal of my own oedipal feelings was the primary difficulty I had to deal with. Whatever fears I had aside, the patient proved to be quite sturdy, and my fears groundless.

In response to my interpretations about her incestuous desires for her father, Mrs. R offered the interesting observation that the man possessed a lower lip that jutted out and that she thought of him as a Ubangi, in other words, as a black man. She was quickly able to see that her rejection of her own son, whom she had imagined to have been fathered by a black man (her father), was actually a rejection or disavowal of her own incestuous desires to have intercourse with her father and to give birth anally to his child.

At this juncture, we were some two and one-half months into treatment. Although it took Mrs. R another two or three years of therapy to work through much of this material, the five-decade-old idea of her son's having been fathered by a black man was essentially resolved at this early phase. Even though much confirmatory material relating to the oedipal nature of the fantasy continued to arise throughout treatment, the intensity of the fantasy abated dramatically and never again caused her to ponder over it or to become depressed about it. The patient was grateful for the relief afforded by this resolution of the symptom. She also condemned Dr. X for his never having probed the relevant issues in depth as we had done. Along with her gratitude, Mrs. R began to experience both a deepening level of erotic feelings for me, as well as an increasing dependency upon me. The analysis of these feelings, along with the understanding of the genesis of her profound rage, occupied the center stage in the remaining years of her treatment.

In a number of dreams following our initial exposition of the oedipal nature of the black man fantasy, Mrs. R was shown as being involved with me in some sort of sexual manner. In one, I was seen as removing her clothes and her dirty undergarments (her guilt over her "black" incestuous wishes) and then was depicted as rubbing her breasts and clitoris in a "loving" sexual manner. She awoke shortly before she might have had an orgasm in a state of combined sexual arousal and anxiety. The anxiety was primarily related to the breakdown of the denial of the incestuous wishes that were evident in the dream. In addition, the idea was expressed that my wife would resent her rivalry for my affection. The obvious underlying oedipal nature of the triadic relationships expressed in these dreams was apparent to both of us, despite the denial so often present in the manifest content of many of these dreams. This was made even clearer in other dreams in which I would be depicted as having the features (the "Ubangi lip," for example) of her father, or where I was seen as her son, who often served as a surrogate for either the father or for me.

In her associations to such dreams, typical apologies were offered by the patient for her having "unseemly" sexual feelings toward me. She also expressed considerable guilt for her renewed masturbation, (discussed later), which now involved the utilization of images and fantasies of me. In addition, however, she began to express increasingly intense feelings of rage toward her former therapist, for his never having explored the incestuous material with her. She also began to verbalize rage toward her father, for having been both provocative and inhibitory with respect to her sexual life. The other men in her life (her dead husband and her son) were also attacked. The latter two were seen as weak and unable to provide her with either sexual or filial gratification. She was furious at her husband's dependency upon his parents (in particular, his tyranical mother) and at his inability to function as a real man with her, either financially or sexually. She likened her son's dependency upon his own controlling wife with her husband's interaction with his mother and raged at the son, too, for his weakness.

Although her denunciations seemed largely justified, a major contributing factor for their appearance soon became manifest. This was her obvious wish to incorporate the phallus of a strong male in order to become more desirable and lovable. This could easily be simply described as "penis envy," but what is more to the point is that the attainment of the idealized phallic self-representation was essentially a means to obtaining the parental (especially maternal) love she had never received as a child. All the men in her life, whether weak or strong, had important attachments to women. Her father had her mother and her husband had his mother, whereas her son had his wife and her former therapist and I had our wives.

Mrs. R, on the other hand, had never had a good relationship with a nurturing female figure. As a result of this deprivation, she was profoundly enraged. In the past, her rage had not generally erupted into her conscious awareness. Rather, she would become depressed. Occasionally, however, the rage would surface and she would become terrified that she might lose the love of the important objects against whom the rage was directed. Both Dr. X and I were protected from this by the development of the erotized transference responses. I have previously described a similar rapidly developing erotized transference response in a patient suffering from lifelong beating fantasies (Myers, 1980).

In one session late in the third year of the therapy, Mrs. R noted that it was the anniversary of her husband's death. She recalled once more how she had elected to visit Dr. X for her session on the day her husband had died, instead of going to visit him at the hospital. She reiterated her guilt feelings over having behaved thus, and then began to describe the warmth and care shown to her by Dr. X over the many years she had seen him.

"You're different than he was. He was friendlier than you are. Besides, you've never really given me what I've most wanted from you. You're probably thinking now that I'm talking about wanting you to sleep with me. That's not really what I meant. What I want most from you is to be held and cuddled by you, to be given to in a way that I was never given to by my husband or by my mother. No one's ever done that for me and no one ever will." With this, she broke down crying and continued to sob until the session ended.

At her next visit, she seemed hesitant to enter the office. I noticed that she was exceptionally well groomed and dressed that day and she began the session by stating that I was going to hate her and would never want to see her again. Her voice had a seductive tone, as if she was almost hoping that I would force her to reveal her thoughts. I finally did enjoin her to tell me what was going on and she reluctantly recounted a dream in which the two of us were lying naked on my couch. We were either in a post-coital embrace or were in a cuddling mode, with great warmth emanating between us. I then directed her mouth to my penis and she began to suck it and my emission came forth in the form of milk for her to nurse on. Suddenly the milk turned sour or ran dry and she furiously bit the head of my penis off and awoke in terror.

Her associations to the dream led from the black man theme, as expressed in the intercourse that preceded the dream on the paternal (black) couch, to the wish to become one with me and/or be nursed by me as a good therapist–mother. The underlying rage at the dry maternal (bad, cold therapist) teat broke through, however, and the anger at the disappointing figures (men, as depicted as phalluses, and mother as depicted as breast and/or phallus) in her life was expressed in the biting off of the head of my penis–breast.

The incorporation of the phallus in order to achieve the idealized phallic self-representation that would lead to being loved by the rejecting parental figures was also contained in this violent gesture in the dream. The reasons for her reluctance to enter my office and to reveal the true nature of her profound narcissistic rage were clearly revealed in the dream and in her subsequent associations to it. We were later able to see that the biting off of my phallus was also an attempt to incorporate my youth and to thereby protect herself from death, which she greatly feared.

As more and more of Mrs. R's profound pre-oedipal yearnings, and the attendant rage underlying them, were revealed and worked through, it became possible for her to achieve a warmer and more loving relationship with her son, in the sense that she no longer expected him either to supply her with the missing phallus she had desired in the past or to provide her with the missing maternal breast to nurture her with and to help keep her alive. She verbalized acceptance of the idea of her own death, because she had finally "lived" (in other words, felt nurtured).

In addition, Mrs. R became more involved with her younger brothers and their families and formed new and meaningful friendships with neighbors, which greatly enhanced the quality of her life. Although she was unable to find a sexual partner, she was able to regularly masturbate to orgasm. She did this, most frequently utilizing fantasies of sexual interactions with me. The guilt feelings engendered by this practice in the past were markedly diminished. The intensity of her erotic feelings toward me lessened slightly, as the underlying rage was revealed and she no longer felt the need for her biweekly sessions. She would return every four to six weeks for a visit and seemed quite happy with the less than absolute termination arrangement we both agreed upon.

At this juncture, I would once more like to mention some of the important points illustrated by this case. Perhaps the most obvious fact in Mrs. R's treatment was the ready accessibility to consciousness of important psychodynamic material. Even more important was the ability of the patient, a woman in her early 70's at the beginning of her therapy with me, to work with this material and with the transference responses developed toward me in a psychoanalytic mode.

Cases like that of Mrs. R should, once and for all, lay to rest Freud's dictum that patients past the age of 50 are not amenable to psychoanalytic types of intervention. Although Mrs. R was hardly in a classical psychoanalysis, she was able to perform many of the functions expected of the younger psychoanalytic patient. She was able to free associate and was also able to work through the transference and resistances that developed to their genetic and dynamic roots. She also worked easily with dreams and fantasies and was able to recover childhood memories. Whether or not she might have been able to undergo a classical analysis at her age is debatable. What seems more important, however, is that she was able to resolve a symptom that had plagued her for nearly five decades. She was also able to achieve both a greater degree of sexual gratification and to improve her relationships with the important objects in her life. These, of course, would be seen as salutory results in any analysis (or in any other form of treatment).

Another important feature in her case was the understanding of the nature of the transference responses. The erotized transference feelings of the patient were ultimately seen to screen off immense rage to depriving parental (particularly maternal) objects. Although this particular transference response is hardly pathognomonic for older individuals, it is important to underscore here that older patients are capable of producing as intense transference responses to their therapists as are younger ones. Although I was prominently seen as the patient's father or as her son in the early phases of the treatment, I ultimately came to be seen as the depriving maternal figures so evident throughout her life. Again, the plasticity and mutability of the transference responses, which we expect in younger patients, was quite evident in this older woman.

7

A FAILED PSYCHOTHERAPY IN A NARCISSISTIC MAN:
Professor F

Professor F, a 60-year-old academician and chairman of the university's department in his particular subject, was referred to me by an internist because of impotency problems of approximately 10 years duration. His difficulties began shortly after his 50th birthday, when he contracted infectious hepatitis. He was hospitalized for six weeks and then experienced moderate to marked debilitation for almost a year. During the period of recovery, his usually rather high level of interest in obtaining sexual gratification diminished dramatically. The change was particularly noticeable in terms of his relationship with his wife, whom he had married at the age of 31.

Mrs. F, a reserved woman, had always waited for her husband to approach her sexually. In the period after his illness, his approaches became less and less frequent, and even these approaches were marred by his occasional failure to achieve an erection. There was a tacit agreement between the couple to blame these difficulties on the sequelae of the illness, but as they became more and more frequent over the ensuing years (especially after Professor F returned to work), it became more difficult to blame the hepatitis for the potency problem.

In his extramarital relationships, which had always played a prominent part of his sexual life, the professor's potency fared somewhat better. His affairs were conducted unbeknown to his wife and were generally casual, with little real emotional outlay being invested by either party. In his youth, he had ranged rather far and wide in his choice of sexual partners. By the time he had reached middle age, however, the women were generally considerably younger than his wife and were either divorced and employees of the university or graduate students who admired Professor F's expertise in their joint field of academic endeavor. Up until the time he contracted hepatitis, he had never experienced any impotency in either his marital or extramarital life. Even after the hepatitis, although he feared that he might have problems in achieving erections with his extramarital partners once he had experienced this problem with his wife, such episodes of impotency occurred rarely.

Professor F's fear of impotency, however, continued to remain with him with each new woman and was one of the major determinants in his seeking out therapy with me. He had seen a psychiatrist for a few visits some 10 years before and had been reassured that the difficulty would soon pass. Since the doctor had not suggested any extensive psychotherapeutic arrangements and since Professor F had no great faith in the efficacy of therapy to begin with, he decided not to pursue the subject further until he was finally pressured into so doing by his wife's complaints to him about his inattention to her sexually when he failed to approach her for months at a time.

The professor was the elder of two children from a wealthy midwestern Protestant family. Both his parents had died when he was in his late 20's and his sister, three years his junior, was not particularly close to him. The only real communication between the two consisted of holiday and birthday telephone calls. Later in the therapy, I came to discover that one of the important determinants in the patient's choice of his wife as a mate was his awe of her famous father, an academician who had written several treatises that had revolutionized his field of endeavor. Here was a more than fitting replacement for his own lost father, a successful businessman with no particular aptitude or interest in academic pursuits. The professor's mother was a housewife, a rather reserved woman whom the patient recalled as never having conveyed any real sense of warmth to him. The patient's two children, a boy of 27, and a girl, 25, were both married. They too, lived in distant cities and would visit Professor F and his wife at either Thanksgiving or Christmas with their spouses and children. The professor saw these clan gatherings as being relatively pleasant occasions, but the thought often crossed his mind that he might prefer to be skiing or lying on a beach than to be bouncing his grandson on his knee.

In discussing his academic career, Professor F spoke about his accomplishments in a rather offhand manner, as if they did not really matter very much to him. Although he was aware that he was well regarded in his field, he had no illusions that he had produced any truly significant corpus of work during the course of his life. Similarly, although he was on a first-name basis with many of his colleagues at his own university, and in a score of other institutions of higher learning, he quite readily confided to me that he did not really think of any of these people as being true friends, nor did he imagine that they regarded him as being such.

When I first saw the patient in consultation, I felt pleasantly disposed toward him because of his ready affability and charm, his elegant choice of words, and his overall handsome, youthful appearance. He certainly gave the impression of being a man considerably younger than his stated age of 60, a man one might readily engage in treatment. But as the number of evaluative sessions increased, I began to have the feeling of talking with a phantom, a man made up of spaces and shadows, a man lacking real substance. The absence of any genuine sense of regard for anything or anyone (including himself) currently impacting on his life worried me. My presumptive diagnosis was that of a narcissistic personality disorder, although I briefly held out some hope that the neurotic depressive elements might be the predominant ones in the picture. This latter hope of mine was, I believe, a fantasy based on my wish to block out my hostile countertransference feelings toward the patient because of his obvious characterological problems, the likelihood of his being difficult to work with or even unanalyzable, and his generally indifferent response to both me and the field of psychiatry. Unconsciously, I also wished to repeat my successful "rescue" of Mr. T, and the fact that this was unlikely to occur with Professor F frustrated me and was initially denied by me.

Despite my reservations about the nature of Professor F's object-relationships, his apparent devaluation of both me and the field of psychiatry, and his lack of regard for introspective processes, I suggested to him after several consultative sessions that he enter psychoanalysis. I mentioned that this approach might best help us uncover the latent factors behind his potency difficulties. In addition, I felt that he could not be reached by more superficial techniques.

Professor F rejected my suggestion, on the grounds that the large increment of time involved would interfere with his heavy teaching and writing schedules. When I inquired as to whether he had other reservations about analysis besides those already mentioned, he denied any. My impression, however, was that he was not only skeptical about the practical results of analysis, but was fearful of submitting to the process. When I asked him specifically about the fears he might have regarding the process, however, he again denied any such concerns. I might add here that I later came to believe that another reservation was that it might seriously interfere with his freedom in continuing his extramarital relationships. He did, however, agree to my next suggestion that he enter into a twice-weekly psychotherapy.

From the very beginning of the therapy with Professor F, it was apparent that he was having considerable difficulty in free associating. If I was relatively silent, little data were elicited in the sessions. Whereas he might talk of his fears of impotency, he would do so in a stereotyped manner with little real deepening of the material. If I dealt with his frequent silences as resistance to revealing his thoughts and feelings, he seemed genuinely perplexed, as if I were speaking to him in some alien tongue.

"No," he would say, "I'm not really holding anything back from you. I just don't know what more to talk to you about. I can repeat what I've said about my life, I mean particular aspects of it, if you wish, but I simply don't know what is significant and what is not. I believe that it would be more productive if you would just ask me specific questions, ones you think are important. In that way, we would probably make more headway than we're making right now."

When I would point out, at such a juncture, that he sounded irritated, again the response was the ubiquitous denial. After a while, I came to agree somewhat with the professor's self-evaluation. In a certain sense, he did not know what to talk about. Perhaps a more reasonable way of stating this would be to say that he was unconsciously fearful of allowing himself to talk about anything that did not appear to be directly goal related. Thus, his need to control his associations paralleled his attempts to control his erections with his wife, a correlation I mentioned to him and one that he acknowledged to be a reasonable sounding observation. Unfortunately, such observations had little more than an intellectual quality for both of us, and no new material would emerge as a result of such interpretations.

I finally came to recognize that I was making too many of these "intellectual" interpretations to the patient. I believe that I was doing this in order to mask my own feelings of boredom and irritation with him for his lack of productivity. In this sense, I realized that I was feeling much the way his wife must be feeling with him, sexually. My understanding, however, changed little. Rather than trying to change the pattern of intellectual interpretations, I persisted with these for a considerable period of time.

The patient was not especially conversant with his dream and fantasy life and any questions from me concerning these areas, elicited a patronizing smile and a simple "No, I haven't had any recently that I can recall." The only subject matter spoken of with any relish at all was that dealing with his rather elaborate plans for upgrading a flagging relationship with a current mistress or for beginning a liaison with a new one. When I questioned him about whether he was feeling depressed or whether he was experiencing any of the somatic symptoms of this syndrome, he would deny the presence of such feelings.

Probably the only negative feelings that were readily acknowledged by Professor F were his feeling upset or irritated, or occasionally even being concerned over his continued state of impotency in his sexual relationship with his wife. Shortly after the beginning of the treatment with me, he had approached his wife for the first time in many months and the attempt had failed, in the sense of his being unable to achieve an erection. It was another month before he approached her again, and this attempt, too, resulted in a frustrating failure for the patient.

As I listened to him describe the attempts with his wife and the feelings pursuant upon his failures to achieve an erection, it became quite clear that he was not especially desirous of having intercourse because of any real interest in her, sexually. Rather, he seemed more intent on achieving an erection in order to satisfy her needs and demands, so that she would be "off his back" and he would be free to pursue his extracurricular interests.

When I inquired as to the specific circumstances surrounding the most recent episodes of sexual failures with his wife, Professor F casually mentioned that his wife had had a hysterectomy a year or two before he had been stricken with hepatitis and because of complications following the procedure, she had received a rather disfiguring surgical scar. In inquiring about this, I was told that she had asked him on a number of occasions whether the scar had produced any sense of revulsion in him and whether he wanted her to undergo plastic surgery. He had assured her that this was not necessary.

When I attempted to pursue the matter further with questions about his associations to the scar, reasoning to myself that the scar might represent some concretization in his mind of the idea of female or male castration, thereby arousing anxiety in him that would unconsciously interfere with his capacity to perform sexually, I met with a dead end. As was typical in Professor F's response to such questions from me, nothing further was forthcoming. Although it was apparent that he was not simply withholding material from me, but rather was unconsciously fearful of associating to the material that had already been brought forth, it was still frustrating to deal with him.

On those occasions when I would attempt to deal with what seemed to me to be references in his speech to transference feelings about me, I would also draw "blanks." He would politely inform me that he had no specific feelings about me. Again, although I recognized the defensive quality of his not allowing himself to acknowledge consciously my importance to him in any manner, it gave us very little to "grab onto" in a psychotherapy geared, as it so clearly was by virtue of his anxiety, to simply attempting to relieve a specific symptom, his impotency with his wife, without allowing us the freedom to modify the rest of his personality.

As the constraints upon the treatment became more and more evident, I pointed them out to the patient repeatedly and once more suggested to him that we widen the scope of the therapy by switching over to a conventional psychoanalysis. At this point, I had a great many reservations about his suitability for analysis, but I also felt that without removing the restrictions laid upon the treatment, we were likely to founder in relatively short order. Needless to say, my suggestion was also motivated by my desire to block out my feelings of hostility to the patient by artificially attempting to add a note of optimism to the outcome by a change to a more demanding therapeutic procedure. Professor F, however, once again rejected the idea of an analysis.

As my frustration with the course of the treatment grew, I once more found myself acting out my unconscious identification with the patient's anxieties about his state of passive helplessness vis-à-vis his problem. When I noticed that I was becoming more active in my pursuit of pertinent psychodynamic factors that might have a bearing on his symptom of impotency, almost directing the sessions into a question and answer type of format, I came to realize how I had identified with his passive, impotent state. I interpreted this to the patient, noting that through the medium of his having limited the scope of the treatment to a symptom-oriented type of therapy, he had unconsciously managed to limit my efficacy as a therapist, perhaps in an unconscious attempt to communicate to me his helpless feelings, with the result that I would thus share his impotency.

Again my somewhat "irritated" interpretive effort fell upon deaf ears. "No doctor, I assure you that I have no desire for you to feel that way. I'm quite sorry that you do. Quite to the contrary, it would be against my own best interests to have you functioning at anything less than one hundred percent of your capacity."

During the course of the more active question and answer type of sessions in which I engaged Professor F, a number of interesting psychodynamic factors relevant to the impotency did emerge. When we spoke in greater detail about Professor F's own parents, it was evident that his mother had been a cold, distant person. Her only means of even remotely offering affection took the form of verbal praise for his superior academic performance. His father would occasionally "rough house" with him when he was a child, which the patient had found enjoyable, but he too, grew rather distant from Professor F when the patient's academic interests drew him further away from the possibility of entering the father's business. Why the patient went in this direction never became clear, despite my repeated efforts to get him to talk about it.

Only with his father-in-law, whom he saw often during his yearlong courtship of his future wife, did the patient find a true warmth. Not only was his father-in-law a remarkable academician, he was also a warm individual. He was a man who had been adored by his daughter, Professor F's wife, until he committed the one major indiscretion of his life, that of having an affair with a younger colleague. The affair was discovered by Professor F's wife shortly before her marriage to the patient. In a dramatic emotional confrontation with her father, she extracted his promise that he would never see his mistress again. She, in turn, promised to keep the matter secret from her own mother, which she did during the 10 years before her mother's death.

The confrontation between father and daughter led to a considerable cooling off of their relationship, which the patient personally experienced as a rather tragic loss. When his father-in-law died, shortly after the onset of Professor F's hepatitis, the patient cried for perhaps the only time in his memory, in response to any conventionally sad occurrence. Not even at his own parents' funerals, had he shed tears. When he looked over at his wife, however, he felt her evident disapproval of his conduct and he dried his eyes. In the 10 years since the funeral, he never cried again. Consciously, he said, he rarely thought of his father-in-law. When I tried to connect his wife's evident critical attitude at his showing an emotional response to his father-in-law's death and his need to deny any feelings of loss toward me over weekend or holiday separations during the limited period of our therapy (in total, it lasted somewhat less than one year), he again smiled patronizingly and denied any such connection.

In conjunction with the material about the confrontation between the patient's wife and her father over the father's affair, and the subsequent profound devaluation of the man in her eyes, the obvious parallel to the patient and his affairs seemed apparent. I wondered if he might be attempting to unconsciously repeat the situation, which he denied. In this one instance, however, he was able to see that he was extremely susceptible to any possible criticisms related to his wife's rigidly judgmental value system. He was able to recognize that she paralleled his own mother in the extreme rigidity of the ego ideals she espoused, and for perhaps the only occasion during the course of the therapy, he was able to resent his wife.

When I inquired as to whether he might impart any of these feelings to his wife (a rather directive suggestion from me, which came up toward the end of the treatment), he was thoughtful for a while and then replied that he might do just that. When I asked him in the next session what had happened, he spoke of relaying a muted-down version of his anger to his wife. She surprised him by acknowledging the correctness of his feelings and even spoke of her regret at having so devalued and alienated her father, whom she had quite genuinely loved. In this setting of rapprochement, the patient once again attempted to have intercourse with his wife and for the first time in many months, he was able to achieve a partial erection.

The salutory result described above was not, however, a lasting one and my wishful expectation that Professor F might now become interested in deepening his exploration of the psychodynamic factors involved in his impotency and in his life was never fulfilled. Perhaps this was also related to his wife's inability to modify her value judgments. Or perhaps it stemmed from his continuing problem in expressing negative feelings to her. To have done so, seemed to me to imply to the patient a real commitment to making their relationship work. This was not one of the results he had bargained for in treatment. His unconscious fears of destroying women, evident in his anger to his wife and his mother, necessitated Professor F's keeping them at a distance, as he did with his wife and his paramours. Consequently, when Professor F's next attempt at intercourse with his wife resulted in impotency, he simply slipped back into a liaison with one of his former mistresses.

One more psychodynamic factor of interest is worth mentioning. This has to do with the professor's sensitivity to aging, especially as manifest in his special awareness of changes with time. In our discussions, it appeared that one of the important determinants of the prolonged response he had suffered after the hepatitis years before had to do with his having reached the age of 50. He could no longer think of himself as a young man. The eventuality and the reality of getting older, of facing debilitating diseases (such as the hepatitis) and even confronting death (so shortly before dramatized in the demise of his father-in-law), had pressed strongly upon his conscious awareness. Although it is likely that aging and death both represented reality fears, per se, they also seemed to quite prominently symbolize castration for the patient. This equation of death and castration is discussed in a later chapter.

When Professor F entered treatment with me, he had reached another momentous age, 60. He spoke of being fearful of losing his good looks and his facility in conquering women sexually as he got older. This was verbalized in lieu of talking of his fears of death, either his own or of the death of any of the significant objects in his life. He also feared that, with advancing age, his potency would totally desert him. When his fears of impotency had abated because of the resumption of relations with his current mistress (after the final failure to achieve an erection with his wife), and when his wife's demands for sexual intercourse became less strident, his need for continuing in treatment with me dissipated. By that time, he had passed his 61st birthday and the decadal milestone that had so upset him had faded from his consciousness. We finally agreed to terminate the treatment, with the proviso that he might return at any time.

At this point, let me underline some of the salient features of this case. It seems prudent to start with the fact that Professor F had very little actual motivation to effect a real characterological change. His prime concern was for symptomatic relief, and really nothing more. In addition, a strong factor in his beginning therapy with me had to do with his wife's finally verbalizing her dissatisfaction with his performance in meeting her rather minimal sexual demands.

What I am attempting to emphasize is that symptomatic and external pressures prompted the patient to seek out help, rather than any internal recognition of the need for change. In this sense, he differed markedly from the five patients described earlier. I believe that his motivational factors would have been poor, regardless of his age at entering therapy. In addition, he had very little respect for the field of psychiatry, as illustrated by his skepticism of its ability to effect any real personality change. Although this may very well have subserved unconscious defensive functions, I believe that this factor, too, should be considered in evaluating his capacity for change.

Another important feature of Professor F's case was his prominent difficulty in obtaining pleasure in any area of his life. Although he could achieve sexual gratification, most particularly in his extramarital affairs, there was little in the way of sharing and higher level object-relatedness involved. What seemed most prominent was a functional pleasure in his ability to perform as a man, rather than the pleasure contained in the interaction between one human being and another. This problem in object-relations pervaded his life, affecting his relationship with his sister, his wife, his children, and his colleagues. I have rarely found patients with such overriding difficulties in experiencing any real pleasure in any facet of their lives to be analyzable. Such difficulties pose profound problems for patients in any form of psychotherapy, as well, regardless of their age.

Also unlike the other five patients, Professor F had minimal contact with his unconscious life and fantasies. He was not conversant with his dreams and seemed caught up in his stream of thought with the day-to-day machinations involving his interactions with his mistresses. Introspection and psychological mindedness were not important features of his personality.

My suggestion that he undergo psychoanalysis was ill-advised, regardless of whether it had been accepted or not. He also had little contact with his emotional (affectual) life, and only on the one occasion, when he recognized his feelings of resentment to his wife for her judgmental qualities, did he exhibit insight into this dimension of his feeling state. This incapacity to recognize and to experience affect would also have been a stumbling block in the path of any possible therapeutic change in either psychoanalysis or psychotherapy.

8
ASSESSMENT OF GENERAL TREATABILITY IN THE OLDER PATIENT

In reviewing the six cases presented here, I want to discuss the general factors, applicable to patients of any age, that affected their capacity to be analyzed, as well as the factors that are only important in patients over 50.

THE LITERATURE

Freud (1905a) felt that being older, in and of itself, was an insuperable obstacle to the analytic process because of the amount of material to be worked through and because of what he felt was an inelasticity of the mental processes of older people. My case material, and that of others noted before, is at variance with these ideas.

Abraham (1919) overcame Freud's injunctions against treating older patients. From his clinical experience, he suggested that treatment failures with such individuals resulted from their reluctance to talk of their instinctual lives, whereas successes were related to the length of the period of good sexual and social functioning the patient had experienced after puberty.

Although many older patients can talk of their sexual lives in considerable detail (as, for example, Professor F), this may have only a limited effect on their ultimate capacity to be analyzed. In addition, some patients (such as Mr. T, Mrs. N, Ms. B, and Mrs. R), who had not had a high level of sexual functioning for long periods in their lives, may be able to achieve much better levels of sexual functioning in later life, as a result of treatment.

Alexander (1944) assessed analyzability in the older patient in terms of the individual's capacity to respond to the trial interpretations offered by the therapist. This can be re-stated as follows: Individuals who exhibit psychological mindedness and introspective capacities seem to be better candidates for analysis. This is, of course, true, regardless of the age of the patient.

Grotjahn (1951) and Meerloo (1953) suggested that aging, rather than hindering analysis, might actually facilitate the process, by virtue of the effect of reality upon long-standing defenses. This is particularly true in the case of narcissistic personalities or in patients with prominent narcissistic defenses. It is not always easy, however, to evaluate whether or not this has happened to an individual. One way, as noted in my description of the evaluative phase with Mr. T, is to ask the patient about the disparity in his presentation in his current sessions and in his previous psychotherapy. What may emerge from such a question is an estimation of a change in motivation, which may be traced to the erosive effect of reality on the individual's narcissistic grandiosity.

Erikson's (1959) concept that the achievement of integrity is one of the prime tasks of the mature individual is of interest with respect to the idea of evaluating analyzability. The more one can accept one's life and one's significant objects, without rage or envy toward them, the more one is apt to be found to be analyzable, regardless of age. In the older individual, what is of particular importance is the assessment of envy directed by the patient toward his children or his younger colleagues. If this is too great, as in the case of Professor F, then the patient is unlikely to be analyzable. Klein's (1963) thoughts about the interferences posed by envy to successful adaptations to old age fit here. Unfortunately, it is often difficult or impossible to assess correctly the amount of envy a patient possesses during the evaluative phase.

Levin's (1965a) paper details the difficulty some older patients have in investing new objects. The capacity to invest new objects must be evaluated in the consultative phase, in order to determine the potential for achieving a strong enough transference relationship with the analyst. The rapidly observable transference dreams of Mr. T, Mrs. N, and Mr. W, indicated their strong transference potential. Obviously, the patient's capacity for reality-testing is important in the assessment of the psychotic versus neurotic transference potential of the patient.

Jacques (1970) described an interesting feature in his paper, which was further elucidated by Kernberg (1980) in one of his books. Simply stated, both observed that if a patient is able to accept his own imperfections, without globally devaluating his prior accomplishments, there is a diminution of his narcissistic defenses. This is an indicator of the patient's capacity for analysis. I would add here that patients who demonstrate this ability to accept their own imperfections are not as frequently overwhelmed by their envy of others who may be thought to possess narcissistic grandiosity they have lost. Hence, their need to defeat the envied analyst by rendering him impotent to help them is not an insuperable obstacle to the analysis or therapy. Mrs. N and Ms. B both had strong problems in this area, and thus nearly defeated their treatments.

Neugarten's (1970) description of the change some older patients describe in their perception of time (the idea of its being finite, rather than infinite) is, I believe, of great importance in terms of assessing analyzability in the older individual. To be more precise, those patients who do not perceive time as being finite seem to me to be either unanalyzable or more difficult to analyze. One must be able to accept the inevitability of one's death, to some extent, in order to be motivated to change one's life.

In line with the above, Mr. T and Mrs. N were both keenly aware of their aging and of the possibility of death, and this awareness intensified their motivation for analysis, which might not have been there at an earlier age. Professor F, on the other hand, denied the idea of his aging and the possibility of his dying, and this was one of many features that contributed to his being untreatable. I would simply like to note here that Neugarten's reference to the capacity of some older individuals to act as "sponsors" to younger people (children, subordinates) is also an important factor in judging analyzability, as it relates to the titer of envy of the young.

Sandler's (1978) patient demonstrated a considerable malleability during his analysis with her, as manifested in job change, change of mate, transference capacity, etc., but it was apparently not easy to predict this from the initial interaction. King (1980) emphasized the sense of urgency introduced into the analyses of middle-aged patients by the perception of their changed life situations. She sees this as facilitating the formation of the therapeutic alliance, and underscored the idea that such patients perceived the treatment as their last chance to modify their lives. The reality factor, noted before, lends an intensity to the motivation to change, which is a positive feature in assessing analyzability.

Kernberg (1980) emphasized the need of the older patient to complete the mourning of lost objects in their lives. He also underlined the importance of accepting their own lives and love objects without a significant need to devalue them. The capacity to do this is taken as a positive indication in assessing analyzability. The correctness of his views can be seen clearly in the cases of Mrs. N and Ms. B, described earlier. Kernberg notes further that narcissistic personalities who are depressed in mid-life tend to become more accessible to analysis than they may have been at an earlier age, which he ascribes to a weakening of the narcissistic defenses and to an increase in self-awareness and in motivation for treatment.

FACTORS IN THE ANALYZABILITY OF THE PRESENTED CASES

Let me turn now to the case histories of my six patients described in this book. I will mention some of the positive and negative features, vis-à-vis the subject of analyzability in each case. Then I will underline the specific factors related to the age of the particular patients.

In Mr. T's case, the negative factors during the evaluation period included his history of past therapeutic failures. Perhaps another way to state this would be to speak of his lack of involvement in the therapeutic process in his prior attempts at treatment. In addition, his lifelong impotency and his tendency toward somatization were also negative factors, as they indicated a considerable amount of primitive rage.

The family history of a rejecting, emasculating, un-nurturing mother and a passive, unsuccessful, rage-filled father, who was not supportive to the patient's masculinity (although he was capable of offering some nurturing to the patient), was not the most hopeful constellation in which to have developed the capacity for basic trust that is necessary for the analytic process to be effective.

On the positive side was the history of the warm, nurturing relationship Mr. T had developed with his childhood sweetheart, L, and with her loving family. In addition, there is the record of success in his army and business careers, which indicated his ability to express aggression and to compete with other men.

When we turn to the area of object-relationships, we note that Mr. T did attempt to satisfy his wives and his other paramours sexually, even if, in some measure, this was done to avoid feelings of humiliation and emasculation. If we couple this with his ability to empathize with his first wife's suffering, when she believed that their sexual dysfunction was due to her ineptitude or her lack of attractiveness, and his consequent admission to her that his problem with erectile impotence had antedated their relationship, we readily recognize that he had a capacity to relate to objects on a post-ambivalent level. This spoke well for his ability to be analyzed.

Mr. T's demonstrable fondness for fine food, his wife, and travel also was evidence of a continuing capacity for pleasure, which boded well for analytic success. His expertise in playing poker, where he could also allow himself to successfully compete with other men, also attested to this ability.

Among the more important positive features in Mr. T's case were his sense of urgency for change and his ability to develop and to recognize the transference (as seen in the dream during the evaluative phase of being rescued from quicksand by my helping hand). I see both of these factors as being specifically related to his age. He clearly stated during the evaluative phase that his motivation for treatment had been given a tremendous impetus by virtue of his nearing 60, the age of his father at his death. He also mentioned his desire to be happier in his life than his father had been.

Although Mr. T was clearly competitive with his father and with me, he was not an intensely envious man. This also stood him in good stead in allowing him to be analyzed and particularly, to be analyzed by a younger man. My relative youth, if anything, allowed him hope, rather than envy. In fantasy, he might borrow from it, not steal from it or from me, in order to be stronger. Although this factor of a relative lack of envy in this patient is not a specific one for determining the capacity of an older individual to be analyzed, it should be apparent that an analysis will not progress well in a person in this age range when too great a titer of envy is present.

In Mrs. N's case, the negative features are more prominent, than in Mr. T's. Her presenting symptom of alcoholism with blackouts can only be seen as a serious negative indicator for analysis, as can her underlying state of depression and her wish for death and for reunion with lost love objects (as, for example, in her identification with her alcoholic mother and her alcoholic older brother), as inferred in the early evaluative phase.

Another negative feature was her rather consistently negative self-image. In addition, her perception that life had not been fair to her indicated a degree of self-pity and a conceptualization of herself as a passive participant in the events of her own life. Other negative factors include the errant quality of her parental input and the absence of an important love object in her life.

Turning to the positive side, one obvious plus for Mrs. N was her evident capacity for empathy, as in her not drinking when she was with her surviving brother. This also demonstrated an ability to relate to objects on a post-ambivalent level. She showed this capacity for high level object-relatedness in her long-standing relationships with several women friends and in the past history of solid object ties with her husband and her son.

Mrs. B also displayed a continuing ability to obtain pleasure, as when she played a good game of tennis. Her dream of reaching out for someone also spoke of a wish to form new object ties, which could be taken to indicate a capacity to form a solid transference relationship with me. Her mourning dream, with its transference allusion during the evaluative phase of the treatment, also demonstrated her access to unconscious material and her ability to work with an analyst through transference. Her specific association to the dream, in which she expressed the desire to become the captain of her fate, was also a positive feature, inasmuch as it indicated a wish to gain control over her chaotic life.

Once again, as with Mr. T, a final factor of great importance in assessing her capacity to be analyzed was related to her age itself. By virtue of having reached an age that was close to that at which her mother had died of alcoholism, her desire to change herself and her life had increased. Although she may also have wished to die and to be reunited with her mother, the stronger desire was to live and to achieve a solid degree of separation from the identification that threatened to swallow her up.

Moving on now to Ms. B's case, a number of negative features stood out quite clearly. First and foremost was the difficulty entailed in assessing the depth of her masochistic need to punish herself and to circumvent any treatment endeavor she might enter (via the proverbial negative therapeutic reaction). The fantasy of having been responsible for her mother's death by being born, was difficult to combat, as were the lesser transgressions she had presumably inflicted upon her father and grandmother. Coupled with the guilt and masochism was the problem of evaluating the intensity of her rage and whether it would predispose her to a transference psychosis, not a transference neurosis. Her history of depersonalization at her father's funeral worried me in this regard, as I saw it as a defensive distortion of her ego functions to ward off her perception of her intense rage.

The obvious parental deprivation was another negative feature in the evaluation of her capacity to form a solid transference relationship. In addition, her obvious reticence about entering into relationships with men throughout her life, based as it was on the fantasy of the feared retaliation by the dead mother if she were to bear a baby herself, bespoke of profound difficulties in this sphere.

On the positive side, however, was the knowledge that Ms. B had had some significant nurturing figures in her life. There was the grandmother and a number of the young farm-girl housekeepers, in addition to the surrogate mother-teacher and the teacher's husband. The ties with the latter pair had been deep, indicating that her capacity for object-relationships had not been all that impaired. This was further demonstrated in the number of close relationships she maintained with women friends and colleagues throughout her life.

In addition, her work life had been a happy, productive one. This led me to believe that her need for punishment was not global and that it could be modified in analysis. She was a fine teacher and a capable artist and she was able to take pride and pleasure in the work of her pupils, which indicated a relative lack of envy vis-à-vis younger people.

Ms. B also had a considerable amount of courage and resiliency. She had stood up to her father, and looked him in the eye, when discussing her career plans with him prior to embarking for college, and she was able to make a break from her home and remaining family ties when she moved to New York. She also handled major surgery (her hysterectomy) alone.

It is in this latter area, the handling of the hysterectomy, that I think a very important factor about Ms. B emerges, which has considerable bearing on assessing her ability to be analyzed. It was as if she had decided, in having the hysterectomy and the hymenotomy, that she had suffered enough, that the debt to her mother had been paid off. Obviously this was not true, as became manifest in the analysis, but the unconscious change in the balance of forces, manifest in the decision to have the latter surgery was an important factor in allowing her to be analyzed. Somehow Ms. B had to reach a reasonable age (over 50) to allow herself to give up the idea of childbearing and to consent to getting on with her life and with her sexual pleasure. Her wish to be "opened up" above (her mind) and below (her sexuality) spoke of a desire to expand her life. I do not believe that she could have done this at a younger age.

In Mr. W's case, the most negative feature was his intense passivity. This was manifest, for example, in the idea that I was to give him my new prop to replace his old, wornout one and in his apathetic approach to seeking out new jobs and new women to enliven his life. The rigidity of his character structure, seen in his persistent use of the airplane imagery, was also a negative feature in assessing his capacity to be analyzed. Another such feature was his very lack of physicality, as evidenced by the difficulty he had in touching people he was close to (which was, in part, responsible for his having pushed his wife away from him and into the arms of their friend). This was obviously related to the lack of physical warmth so apparent in his relationships with his distant parents.

Mr. W had also had a heart attack several years before and one could question the wisdom of embarking upon a probing course of treatment in a man with proven coronary artery disease. But one could question the wisdom of such a course of therapy in a patient of any age.

In turning to the positive features in his case, although he may have been passive, Mr. W had also demonstrated that he had been active enough to fly one hundred combat missions over Europe, to marry and to father a family, and to help run a major company. In other words, he had been a successful man, whose view of his life had been positive until the series of negative events that occurred ultimately brought him into analysis.

His freedom in bringing up unconscious material (his dream, for example, during the evaluative phase) and his ability to associate to the dream and to my interventions, made me feel that he would be able to free associate in analysis with relative ease. He was also able to handle the early transference allusions I made, without balking. This, too, seemed a positive feature in assessing his capacity for being analyzed.

Mr. W was also a man who had maintained a number of very close object ties throughout his life, despite the series of staggering blows he had suffered prior to seeking help. Although he spoke of feeling distant from his family, they never ceased to maintain consistent ties with him, as did his friends.

What seemed most related to his age, however, was the feeling that he had no other choice, but to seek help and to try to trust me. He was clearly a man who would not have sought out treatment (a rather negative feature, in the sense of his willingness to depend upon another human being), had he not been desperate. He obviously wanted to derive something more from his life than he was deriving, before he died. This probably would never have arisen as a motivating factor, had his wife not left him. I cannot specifically relate this to older age, but job loss, object loss, and ill health are clearly problems of this age period that are not quite as common in the younger years. Hence, once more, the impetus to achieve some modicum of happiness before death was one of the prime motivating factors in pushing Mr. W for treatment and in making him a better analytic risk than he would have been at an earlier period in his life.

If we turn now to Mrs. R, we can see that there were a number of rather negative factors in her past history in evaluating her capacity to be analyzed or to be treated by analytic psychotherapy. For one thing, her mother was a cold, ungiving, narcissistic woman who was always highly critical of the patient. The father, although warm toward her prior to her adolescence, became vituperative toward her after she became a sexual being (despite his own rather blatant exposure of his own sexual relationships with the mother).

In addition, we have the patient's lifelong quasi-delusional idea of having been impregnated by a black man, and her difficulties in being close to her son. A competent analyst had treated her for two decades, and had opted to give her electroconvulsive therapy, rather than to probe her psyche in an analytic mode. Finally, she had demonstrated a rather limited capacity for object-relationships during her life, although she had maintained a number of friendships with women she had worked with.

On the positive side, she demonstrated ready access to psychodynamically laden unconscious material, without any discernible disorganizing effect on her personality. She also gave ample evidence (perhaps too ample) of an easy capacity to develop a transference relationship, with both erotized and ambivalent features being demonstrable quite early in treatment. She was able to free associate and had ready access to dreams and early memories.

Furthermore, Mrs. R demonstrated a healthy degree of independence, in being able to support herself (despite her lack of formal education) in a very agreeable style. She was highly thought of and was asked to remain at work long after the normal retirement age. Once given the evidence of my interest in exploring her difficulties, rather than in suppressing them, she became a willing participant in the therapeutic work.

It is not possible for me to say whether or not Mrs. R would have been such a good patient at any other time in her life, but my presumption is that she should have been given a chance to be. It may be that the freedom from object ties (freedom from a divided loyalty between analyst and husband, as had occurred in her earlier treatment) may have made her therapy with me easier. In this sense, her age may have helped her do as well as she did. This is hard to tell.

Finally, let me examine the case of Professor F. Here, one is hard pressed to find any positive features in the case. Negativity is stamped all over the past history and the evaluative phase of the treatment with this man. It is quite amazing to me, in retrospect, that I persuaded myself that he was at all analyzable.

He had a long history of transient extramarital affairs, characterized by little or no emotional involvement, and a special emphasis on narcissistic gratification (maintenance of the fantasy of the grandiose self). He did not really come for therapy of his own volition, as motivated by any real desire for characterological change, but rather, he came at the behest of his wife, who complained of his inattention to her sexually. He entered therapy primarily for relief from a troublesome symptom, which affected his image of himself, not because of any concern about the effect that the symptom had upon the depth of the relationship with his wife.

Professor F had no faith in the efficacy of the therapeutic process, partly based upon a prior treatment failure. His lack of desire to become therapeutically involved paralleled his lack of involvement in other areas of his life, such as his lack of closeness with his wife, children, sister, colleagues, and work. He expressed the idea that his self-gratification (skiing, affairs, etc.) took precedence over his interactions with objects, such as his grandchildren, or his involvement in treatment. He was not an introspective or psychologically minded man, he had little access to his unconscious processes (dreams, fantasies, etc.), and he had great difficulty in free association. His envy of my youth (clearly a function of his fears of aging, which he equated unconsciously with castration) probably contributed to his unconscious need to render me therapeutically impotent and to thereby triumph over me.

He also demonstrated his lack of empathic object-relatedness by showing no real concern for his wife's feelings with regard to his impotency. He desired potency with his wife simply to get her off his back, so that he might pursue his narcissistically gratifying affairs without her interference. His fear of loss of love objects was so inordinate that he avoided any really meaningful involvement with such objects.

What might have been a positive feature in another individual was a negative one in Professor F. He had a depressive response to decadal milestones, but simply dealt with them by redoubling his narcissistic defenses, rather than by accepting the limitations of age and turning to his important objects for succor. Finally, his lack of real pleasure in any area of his life spoke to a poor capacity for sublimation, another factor of importance in assessing analyzability generally.

SUMMARY

Let me simply note here that I have stressed the impetus given to the desire to change by virtue of getting older and close to death as a positive feature in the capacity of the older individual to be analyzed. I am indebted to Dr. Paul Bradlow (1981) for the suggestion that the accumulated losses of love objects helps the older individual undo his sense of denial about his narcissistic invulnerability (grandiosity) and thereby makes him more amenable to treatment. This is similar to Kernberg's (1980) idea of lifelong narcissistic defenses weakening in older individuals and to King's (1980) idea of the last-chance concept about changing one's character structure.

9

THE IMPACT OF LOSSES ON THE SENSE OF SELF

In this chapter, and in the three chapters that follow, I discuss various developmental problems found in the older patient. In a sense, all the topics to be discussed center around the issue of loss, in one form or another. I will illustrate the broad ideas presented with some clinical excerpts from the cases presented in this volume.

LOSS OF, OR DECREASE IN, ATHLETIC SKILLS

For the individual who has made a considerable narcissistic investment in achieving and maintaining certain athletic skills, the loss or diminution of these skills can be damaging. Changes in athletic ability are seen as signs of aging or of loss of potency or of loss of physical attractiveness. The greater frequency of injuries experienced by many older individuals engaging in active sports can also be alarming.

An example of the above can be found in one of the few affective interchanges I had with Professor F. In describing his reluctance to spend the Christmas holidays with his children and grandchildren, he spoke of his wish to be skiing instead. When I inquired further about his thoughts in this regard, he referred to the exhilaration he experienced skiing briskly down a slope. He mentioned his favorite ski resort longingly, and my own feelings resonated with his, inasmuch as I had joyfully skied the same area on a number of occasions.

When he casually interjected the names of some trails he had enjoyed, however, I was surprised at the particular ones he had chosen. These slopes were gentle ones, not especially apt choices for brisk downhill runs. Without mentioning my familiarity with the area, I asked why he had thought of those particular runs. He became silent and then made a vague allusion to the openness of the trails, clearly evading my question. When I thought of pressing forward with my questions, I realized that I was feeling competitive with the patient and that some narcissistic needs of my own had been aroused, as well as a wish to expose his inadequacy to him. But for one of the few times in his treatment with me, the patient broke through his defensive veneer and exposed his feelings to me.

"I used to ski deep powder all day long," he noted, "but I can't do it anymore. My thighs begin to quiver after about an hour of it, and I have to stop. It's the same thing as sex, I can't go on as long there, too, as I used to. It's not a good feeling. It makes me feel older and used up. I don't like it."

Professor F's confession was accompanied by a genuine expression of sadness, which seemed to show that it was getting harder and harder for him to maintain his facade of youthfulness for himself, let alone other people. The increasing difficulty of this endeavor sorely taxed his self-esteem. I realized that my surge of competitiveness had been based on my own need to deny any decrease in my athletic prowess, for reasons that were not all that far removed from the patient's. The resolution of the countertransference response in me, restored my empathy for the patient and led to a clearer understanding of his need to deny the diminution in his athletic skills.

The loss of self-esteem attendant upon decreases in athletic prowess, was also a significant part of the analyses of both Mrs. N and Mr. W. Mrs. N had been an exceptional tennis player in her youth. When she observed younger women playing better than she did, she felt "put down," "denigrated," and "older." On occasions when she managed to score points with crosscourt smashes, or to record aces with her serve, her self-esteem rose. Similarly with

Mr. W and his squash game. With both patients, the capacity to retain long-standing athletic skills was taken by them as evidence of the permanence of their youthfulness and their sexual attractiveness. Diminution of such abilities was seen as a one-way road leading to a lonely old age, devoid of sexual partners and ultimately culminating in death.

The athletic skills in all three of these patients had either been developed in the context of relationships with important parental objects (their fathers) or were developed in order to impress the parental object (as with Mrs. N and her father). Hence the loss of the skill was seen unconsciously as a further weakening (in fantasy) of an already attenuated object tie. For older individuals, particularly those who have suffered a number of narcissistic mortifications, any factor that diminishes the capacity to measure up to an idealized internalized parental standard reduces their self-esteem, which is often perceived as the loss of an important object.

LOSS OF, OR DECREASE IN, SENSORY ACUITY

One of the sure signs of aging experienced by most people, is the gradual recognition that they need glasses in order to read, and patients frequently respond to this discovery with denial, so as not to diminish their self-esteem.

For Ms. B, the theme of the man with the glasses, which referred back to her sexual fantasies about her beloved teacher's husband, was seen also to relate to her masturbatory fantasies about me. This became apparent after she had noticed that I, too, like the teacher's husband, needed glasses to read with.

"I'm glad that you do," Ms. B said one day, referring to my need for the reading glasses. "I don't have to feel quite so freakish and old for needing them myself. I don't like that feeling. It's not a comfortable one for me. I feel like I've missed enough of the world as it is, because of my neurosis, not to have to miss any more of it because I can't see enough of what's going on around me. Thank goodness I can still hear what people are saying. I'd feel even lousier about myself if I were missing that, too."

In this frank disclosure, the patient revealed her equation of diminished sensory acuity with the process of getting older (seen as being "freakish") itself. The concept of missing something, read as sensory deprivation at one level and as potential object deprivation at another, was a very poignant one for Ms. B., particularly in view of her history of repeated parental deprivations and object losses. Here, vision and hearing are equated with oral organs of incorporation and with the means of ingesting the world of stimuli and of available objects. To be deprived of this was a depressing thought for the patient. In addition, putting on one's reading glasses in front of others was a public announcement of one's aging, and a risk of rejection by potential sexual objects.

The concept of being "freakish" and of "missing" something, also resonated with the patient's feeling of being castrated. The perception of herself as being without the phallus she believed her father prized so highly contributed to her diminished self-esteem, as well as her chronic depression, anger, and feelings of entitlement. All this led to further feelings of depletion. Similar examples of this type of diminution secondary to sensory acuity defects could be seen with a number of my other patients, such as Mr. W. He described his difficulty in picking up the ball in his visual field when playing squash. He typically related this to his youthful flying capacity to easily pick up a German plane in his field of awareness, even in the dimmest light of dawn. The change made him feel older and more unsafe, and neither feeling helped his self-esteem.

LOSS OF, OR DECREASE IN, REPRODUCTIVE AND/OR SEXUAL CAPACITY

Mrs. N and Ms. B had had hysterectomies prior to their analyses with me. Although Ms. B felt freed of a possible retaliation by her dead mother, by virtue of her incapacity to have a baby, she and Mrs. N both experienced the loss of the uterus, and of its baby-growing capabilities, as a sign of getting older and of becoming less sexually attractive to men. To both women, the loss of the uterus was also connected with a fantasy of the loss of the potential for producing new objects, who would be clones of their lost love objects. This was especially true for Mrs. N, who had actually borne a child, the son who had been killed in the Vietnam war.

"Sometimes I feel the way I used to feel before I'd get my period," Mrs. N said one day, around the time of the anniversary of her son's death. "It makes me feel very sad when I get that way. I try to will the hysterectomy scar off of my abdomen, so that I can imagine I'm about to bleed again. If only I could get my periods back, then maybe I could replace him [her son] and protect him this time from dying in that lousy war. I suppose I could also give birth to all of them, my husband, my father, my mother, my brother, all of them. All I need is the capacity to bleed one lousy time a month. It never seemed like such a terrific thing before, when I had it. But now that I don't, the thought of it gets to be so all-consuming. God I feel so inadequate now. As if I've been scarred in some deep place in my soul, and I'll never be able to be whole again."

To Ms. B, the loss of the uterus was seen more as a loss of what was perceived to be the seat of her sexual feelings, a loss she had incurred before she had ever really allowed herself to experience such feelings interpersonally. She felt cheated by the surgery. The fantasy that men would find her defective and lacking without her uterus was one of the many factors that contributed to her opting for a homosexual liaison as a long-term relationship, rather than risking rejection in a heterosexual encounter.

All the male patients I have described here presented with complaints of impotency. They all felt wounded in their self-esteem because of acute or chronic sexual performance difficulties. All three felt "damaged" in the sense of their "maleness," which interfered with their abilities to interact adequately with potential sexual partners. In this sense, their loss of self-esteem contributed to their ongoing object deprivation, which, in turn, further intensified their difficulties.

Loss of sexual potency was frequently equated by all of these men (particularly by Professor F) with the end of their lives, as if sexuality was the central force governing their lives and lending it any and all color and purpose. Perhaps because he had suffered from impotence for the greater part of his life, Mr. T's motivations for obtaining analytic treatment transcended the mere wish for potency, and he was able to remain in treatment for a longer period of time and perhaps to benefit more from the therapy than the other two male patients. This is an important factor in the assessment of analyzability in patients in this age group. That is, that they be able to recognize that they are in treatment for difficulties other than their sexual performance. Their accurate perceptions in this regard seem to imply that they see themselves as more complete (whole) individuals and that they may be able to relate to others on a more complete (higher) level, rather than simply interacting with objects in order to satisfy and gratify sexual or nurturing needs.

Sexuality, per se, is an important part of the lives of older patients. Whether or not analysts wish to deny this, it is true. It seems that the individuals who led active sexual lives (whether interpersonally or masturbatory) in their youth will continue to do so or to want to do so as they grow older.

LOSS OF, OR DECREASE IN, SEXUAL ATTRACTIVENESS

The idea of being perceived as less sexually attractive to a potential sexual (or love) object than one used to be is difficult for most older individuals to deal with. This is especially true for narcissistic individuals, such as Professor F, who have based their lives on their ability to obtain an endless series of modularly replaceable sexual partners at will, to deal with current needs and anxieties. The perceived inability to find new partners evokes a considerable degree of separation and castration anxiety in such patients, as well as an increasingly prominent element of depression. Dysphoric affects such as these may be the primary motivating factors that propel such patients into treatment. The long-standing need to deny any dependency feelings on external objects, which is so typically seen in narcissistic patients, is battered by the realities attendant upon the discovery of a receding hairline and an expanding waistline. Such narcissistic mortifications may increase motivation, to allow an intensive treatment, such as analysis, to be undertaken and successfully completed.

To a great extent, our society encourages narcissistic attempts to deny certain aspects of aging, as when individuals color their hair to remove telltale traces of graying, combat baldness with hair transplants, or remove lines and shore up sagging jowls by plastic surgery. The implicit equation is that youth equals sexual attractiveness.

All the patients described here bemoaned their loss of sexual attractiveness at one time or another. To Professor F, it represented a threat to the accessibility of prospective sexual partners. When his hairline receded, he underwent a painful hair transplant procedure, in order to restore his threatened sense of youthfulness. Exercise routines were common to almost all the patients described. Many hours were spent weekly in tightening up their stomach muscles, so that their bellies would not bulge and give dramatic evidence to the omnipresent inroads of age. "Nobody wants a fat lover" was a frequent refrain.

Of all the patients mentioned, however, none felt the aging of her own body as acutely as Mrs. R. It was more than simply a matter of her actual age that so concerned her. It was rather a question of her having missed out on sexual pleasure for most of her life. Now that she had finally realized her potential in this regard (in an interpersonal sense), she had no partner to pursue her desires with. She was not an unattractive woman. Quite to the contrary. She had a comely face and a nice figure for a woman of her age, but she was in her 70's and the number of men available for her to date was small. The idea that I would never see her as a prospective sexual partner seemed the cruelest humiliation of all, since I was the one who had helped her unearth her buried desires.

Many sessions were spent decrying the ignominious ironies of the aging process. Mrs. R was thrown back upon the need to gratify her own desires through masturbation, a practice she had discarded during her marriage. This made her feel guilty, and intensified her feelings of humiliation because she felt out of control as a result. Her shame and guilt were related back to oedipal fantasies, expressed in current-day transference derivatives toward me. As the treatment progressed, she was later able to masturbate with a minimal amount of guilt and shame and considerable sexual pleasure.

When these patients were able to come to terms with the idea of a decrease in their own sexual attractiveness to others, they often were able to make more appropriate object choices than they had been able to make in the past. The acceptance of their own physical limitations led them to judge prospective partners in a different light than they had done theretofore. Criteria based on deeper, more human values were generally adopted by most of them, with the exception of Professor F. Thus, what was initially seen as a limitation, and was perceived as a blow to their self-esteem, ultimately came to be seen as the stimulus for adopting a new attitude toward potential love objects, which led to a greater return in human interactions.

LOSS OF, OR DECREASE IN, INTELLECTUAL AND COGNITIVE FUNCTIONS

One of the most sobering and depressing occurrences that older individuals experience is a decline in the intellectual functions. This usually manifests itself in episodes of forgetting and difficulties in learning. These malfunctions are then compounded by difficulties in concentration, which are part and parcel of feelings of depression in many of these patients. Worries over the intellectual decline lead to ever-burgeoning feelings of depression, concentration lapses, and a diminution in self-esteem, which add an intense emotional overlay to the underlying organic process.

Patients caught up in this vicious circle see themselves as deteriorating and unattractive. They become irritable and defensive, which tends to alienate them even further from the objects around them and leads to a greater sense of isolation and loneliness.

Because of the frequent phallicization of the intellect, deterioration in mental functions is usually equated with castration. Feelings of being less attractive sexually lead to a withdrawal from important objects and help to promulgate a sense of loss and separation, and attendant anxiety and depression.

Mrs. R frequently found herself forgetting the time of her appointment and would often call me to check the appointed hour. She was ashamed of this sign of "weakness" and felt certain that I would reject her for this "flaw." The intellectual "weakness" and "flaw" were easily related to her perception of herself as castrated, and she used them to reinforce her feelings of being "unworthy" of receiving my sexual attentions. This drove her back upon herself and her masturbatory practices, in order to rebuild her self-esteem in fantasied interactions with me. Unfortunately, for a long while the masturbation itself made her feel ashamed and guilty and also diminished her self-esteem, thus working at cross purposes to the content of the conscious fantasies themselves. Only with the working through of the transference relationship to its genetic roots could the dysphoric affects be ameliorated and the intellectual deficits experienced in their own terms.

When Mr. W first entered the consulting business, he experienced a considerable degree of anxiety because of his long period of enforced inactivity. At first, he had some difficulty remembering the names of some of the people he was meeting for the first time and in grasping the complexities of his new role. Briefly, he imagined himself to be slipping intellectually, but he was able to persevere in his endeavors, overcome his anxieties, and ultimately, convince himself of his intellectual intactness. This belief that he was slipping intellectually had thrown him into a brief "tailspin," with a concomitant downturn in his self-esteem. Again, this was related to a phallicization of his intellectual capacities and to his perception of himself as being castrated after his heart attack and his wife's rejection.

PHYSICAL ILLNESS

The threat of acute or chronic physical illness is ever present in the aging process. Cardiovascular problems, cancer, and a host of metabolic and organ system malfunctions preoccupy many older people. When the preoccupation becomes reality, however, a number of processes occur that are difficult to reverse.

When especially valued organs, such as the heart and the brain, are threatened, patients generally experience an intense castration anxiety. Even when individuals recover from the immediate episode, they are still likely to conceptualize themselves as being diminished sexually. Such individuals often back off from sexual relations with their mates. This sexual withdrawal diminishes both sexual pleasure and prevents positive feedback to self-esteem, and alienation from the mate occurs. As noted, Mr. W underwent just such an experience after recovering from his heart attack, and this contributed to his estrangement from his wife.

Less dramatic illnesses may also lead to profound feelings of depletion and to diminutions in self-esteem in older individuals. In the case of Mrs. R, her bunions enhanced her sense of herself as ugly and unattractive sexually. She was able to relate this to her sense of her genitals as ugly, and to her perceptions of herself as "defective" and "unlovable," since she did not possess the genitals of a man which she felt her parents wanted her to have.

Physical problems also increase feelings of dependency and diminish one's sense of control over the world, which contribute to a diminished self-esteem and to perceptions of oneself as emasculated and impotent. Feelings of depression add to the already existing problems and another vicious circle of defeat, depletion, and depression comes into play.

Thus, in all the areas detailed in this chapter, loss of physical prowess, or of intellectual competence, leads to a loss of self-esteem, and a subsequent alienation from real or potential love objects. This aberration decreases the possibility of obtaining positive feedback from these objects. One of the objectives of analytic treatment with such people is to enable them to accept the physical and mental limitations of aging, to recognize the superficiality of narcissistic values, and to enhance their capacity to relate to the self and the object world in a deeper, more gratifying manner.

10
THE IMPACT OF RETIREMENT

Retirement, whether voluntary or enforced, is a major dislocation for the older individual. This is true whether the job is performed outside the home or whether it involves responsibility for the physical and psychological well-being of growing children. When one's work life comes to an end, changes occur. These may be good or bad, depending upon the individual case, but they cannot be avoided.

In this chapter, I examine some of these changes under two broad categories: stopping work outside the home and the "empty nest" syndrome.

STOPPING WORK OUTSIDE THE HOME

Life Timing and How Work Stoppage Occurred

Much of the response of life changes depends upon whether or not the changes are expected. When individuals work for a corporation and are approaching the age of 65, they can anticipate their retirement. But the same individuals, at age 55, will be taken by surprise if the company goes bankrupt or if they are fired. Although there are certain issues that must be confronted, regardless of whether the event is expected, if it is, it can be gotten used to in advance. If it is unexpectèd, it may overwhelm the individual's ability to deal with the situation, and thereby create a mini-traumatic neurosis.

When individuals leave jobs voluntarily, they usually feel that the situation is under their control. When a person is forced out of a job, for one reason or another, there is a sensation of helplessness. This latter feeling is hardly conducive to the maintenance of a healthy self-esteem.

Among the individuals described in this book, the person who best exemplifies the specific difficulties of forced retirement is Mr. W. As noted, he had been a corporate executive in a successful company for much of his business career. Due to a series of unforeseen and largely unpredictable world events, the company's fortunes had changed and bankruptcy had been declared. Mr. W thus found himself out of work at the age of 58. Fortunately for him, he had been sufficiently resourceful, financially, to have provided himself with enough money to live on for the rest of his life. What he had been unable to provide, however, was the emotional cushion to withstand the sudden change in his life.

"It was as if I'd expended all my energy trying to save the company," Mr. W said. "I didn't have anything left over for myself. I think I must have been wearing blinders or goggles while it was occurring and I didn't take them off until it was too late. Every ounce of my strength went into holding back the stick to keep the plane flying and then it finally went into a stall and I felt as if I were unable to prevent it from crashing. I think I must have blacked out then, the sort of thing that happens in a power dive. Then just when I started to clear my head again, my heart attack came along and I went into another tailspin. I don't recommend it as a steady diet."

What stands out in Mr. W's description of the circumstances surrounding his company's bankruptcy is his sense of helplessness to control the events. His field of vision narrows, making him even more vulnerable to the overwhelming stimuli that threatened him from all sides. Finally, the plane he pilots goes into a stall and threatens to come apart, and he is overwhelmed by overpowering feelings he cannot control. His feeling of himself as a competent man, a leader who guides the company through stormy periods, is shattered. Engulfed by this tide of events, he surrenders to a terrifying passivity (the blackout). His sense of self-worth is dramatically altered, as is his perception of his own body and the world around him.

As Mr. W noted, just as he begins to emerge from the effects of the loss of his job, he has a myocardial infarction. In both our minds, the bankruptcy of his company made his heart attack more likely. And the physical illness pushes him back into the depths from which he had just emerged. His feeling of loss of control over his body intensifies his perception of himself as someone who can no longer control the corporate world he has lived in for the past three decades.

Finally, when his wife divorces him to marry their mutual friend, Mr. W is shattered and it takes years before he can find the strength to seek out treatment. Little wonder that he stops analysis before reaching the goals I had envisioned for him. He opts for the restoration of the feeling of control, rather than for a thorough working through of the transference neurosis.

Redistribution of Drive Energy

Work has frequently been described as a means of sublimating libidinal and aggressive energy. When routine work is terminated, other channels must be found for this energy. If the work stoppage can be anticipated, other avenues of discharge may be sought out in a leisurely manner. These may include volunteer work, hobbies, or travel. Such methods may, for resourceful individuals, simply be a continuation of lifelong interests that developed independently of their work.

When the work stoppage is unanticipated or unwanted, and when no new normal work outlet can be found for those individuals who have not yet reached their self-appointed retirement age, anxiety, depression, and other dysphoric affects interfere with the re-direction of their drive energy. Then, drive derivative fantasies and actions may lead to even more anxiety and other unwanted affects.

Ultimately, such individuals may feel out of control and helpless, passive victims of their passionate drives and affects. Without understanding love objects in their lives to help them with these untoward feelings, the forcibly retired older individual feels emasculated, with a loss of self-esteem.

Mrs. R had inhibited her sexual feelings for much of her life. During the course of treatment, as the black man fantasy came to be understood by both of us as a derivative of her oedipal desires for her father, sexual wishes toward me in the transference came clearly to the foreground. She ardently searched for available objects to interact with, but understandably, it was not easy for a woman in her mid-70's to find an appropriate man. She was forced to gratify her desires through masturbation, with fantasies of sexual liaisons with me. These masturbatory fantasies caused her much shame and guilt for a considerable period of time.

When she retired from the job she had worked at full time until she was nearly 75, she had no readily available channel for the drive energy that had been expended in her work. Even though her retirement had been planned, she was at a loss as to how to spend her time. She had never developed any athletic skills or hobbies, and she had little desire to travel widely. In the time it took her to develop other interests, she felt besieged by the increased intensity of her drives, especially her sexual desires and she felt increasingly angry at being unable to find a man to gratify her. In addition to expressing her apprehensions that I would abandon or reject her for her outbursts of anger and her "unseemly" sexual desires, she also berated me for having helped her to uncover her wishes and then frustrating her in not helping to gratify them.

Mrs. R masturbated more frequently, and became almost compulsive and frenzied on several occasions. Her fantasies centered around violent encounters with men, generally me or some thinly disguised surrogate, in which she was forcibly taken, sexually. During this period, she felt intense shame and guilt, not only for the content of the sexual fantasies, but also the concomitant feeling of being out of control. Similar, though less intense, feelings were expressed by Mr. W in conjunction with some of his own angry masturbatory feelings, prior to his finally linking up with an appropriate heterosexual love object.

In both patients, the adolescent sense of being a passive victim of overwhelming drives permeated their verbalizations. Mrs. R exhibited another adolescent feature, inasmuch as she felt it was "unseemly" for a woman of her age to have such strong sexual desires (the typical adolescent view of parental and grandparental figures). The analyst must be aware of the presence of any significant countertransference responses to upsurges in patients' sexual and aggressive drive derivative fantasies and wishes.

Changes in Object-Relationships

The importance of understanding love objects in the life of an older individual who has stopped working cannot be over-estimated. This is particularly true for those individuals whose job terminations have not been desired. Such people are likely to suffer from strong feelings of self-hatred, which may lead to a need to punish themselves. One unfortunate method employed in such a situation is to alienate the significant objects in their lives.

Alienating a love object, as was seen in the case of Mr. W, is complex and involves many determinants. The increased anger Mr. W felt as a result of his abrupt cessation of work (without an appropriate avenue in which to channel his aggressivity), led to his perception of himself as an unlovable person. In order to protect his wife from his anger, he unconsciously needed to push her away.

When his difficulties were compounded by his myocardial infarction, he became even more dependent on his wife and more negative about himself. His perception of himself as a diminished masculine and sexual figure, led to a further need to push his wife away. When she finally responded to his overt and covert messages by moving toward a liaison with their friend, his perception of himself as an angry, emasculated man increased, and he felt even more depressed and detached. Finally his wife left him, and his level of desperation reached such an intensity that he sought out treatment, an approach that was contrary to his natural philosophical bent.

In an individual such as Mr. W, who views his feelings of dependency as a sign of weakness, the wish to turn to love objects in times of stress may be suppressed. The wish itself is felt to be passive and feminine and is equated with a perception of the self as emasculated. This often leads to a pseudo-independence, which, as noted above, may alienate significant love objects and lead to actual feelings of deprivation and depression.

In other individuals, feelings of neediness and of dependency are all too readily acknowledged. The person in question besieges the available love objects with requests for reassurance and for gratification, often to the point of overwhelming them. This pattern, too, may ultimately alienate the love object and dry up one of the individual's sources of emotional nourishment. In such cases, these people become inordinately needy and dependent patients when they enter therapy, which may anger and alienate the therapist. Repeated rejections by objects leads to a perception of the self as unlovable and to an ever-increasing need for external gratification. Frustration of such demands is often followed by periods of depression.

At periods of crisis in their lives, such as when employment has been terminated, older individuals may turn to their families for aid. This may often mean having to ask their children for help. If the relationship with the children has been a good one, they may be of great support. If it has not, as was initially the case with Mrs. R and her son, the dependency wishes become frustrated and considerable anger builds up toward the child. This leads to guilt and to feelings of self-hatred, which are hard for older individuals to deal with. It also may lead to an envy of the youth of the younger person (the child) and to a concomitant need to compete with and destroy the successes of the child. This, too, leads to considerable feelings of guilt and to feelings of being a "bad" or "unworthy" person. Treatment often enables older patients to mitigate their envy and to view the situation as one in which their narcissistic grandiosity may be displaced onto their children (or child surrogates, such as a younger colleague or a younger analyst). Without treatment, potentially supportive object-relationships may turn sour or be broken off entirely.

Friendships are also likely to be affected by job termination. If the changed status affects the economic potential to keep up with the Joneses, then a narrowing of the social circle may ensue, with attendant feelings of loneliness, isolation, and depression. The very fact of the job termination itself, with its accompanying loss of self-esteem, may lead to withdrawal or defensive posturing with friends, which may lead to difficult or even ruptured relationships. If the job termination is accompanied by physical changes or changes in marital status, as with Mr. W, then even friendships may be shaken, with their possible dissolution. The capacity to form new friendships is strongly limited when an individual is suffering from feelings of diminished self-esteem. This loss of self-esteem affects all old and new object-relationships.

I have spoken of behavior patterns that may create problems in already existing object-relationships. What of the older individual who no longer has significant object-relationships? What becomes of them, when they stop working outside the home? In essence, increased self-hatred and increased neediness and dependency may become even more apparent. With no available objects to meet their needs, these people often feel that they are helpless and that they cannot control their drives, their needs, and the external world. All this contributes to a perception of the self as powerless, emasculated, and beaten.

Analysis or therapy may be the only modality that can be of help to these individuals. It provides a necessary object-relationship (albeit a hired one) on which to displace important libidinal and aggressive drive derivative wishes. The analyst then helps these patients to regulate their drives (as an external adjunct to their egos and superegos) by providing a model for identification (an identification with the analyst's capacity to deal with strong feelings, such as the intense affects involved in the transference, without resorting to action). The analyst also helps the patient deal with self-esteem problems and provides a forum for understanding long-standing difficulties in object-relationships.

Self-esteem Regulation

As has been noted, all the factors previously discussed have an important bearing on the function of self-esteem regulation in the individual, particularly in the older patient. It seems important, however, to underline several of these factors as being worthy of special notice.

In a general sense, whatever allows older individuals to see themselves as being more passive, more dependent, and more helpless than they perceived themselves to be previously, will diminish their self-esteem. An ignominious work termination, debilitating physical illness(es), and disruption by death, divorce, or disharmony of important object-relationships all will contribute.

In addition, an increase in instinctual drive derivatives, leading to serious conflict with the superego or the ego ideal, will increase the sense of helplessness and decrease feelings of self-esteem. Other shame- or guilt-producing feelings, such as envy, will also lead to such changes.

Finding a new job or new life interests, developing new confidence in oneself as a sexual being, by virtue of becoming involved in a new and meaningful object-relationship, or deepening contacts with family and friends, are all ways of ameliorating deficits in self-esteem. Analysis, or analytic psychotherapy, is also very important. When older patients recognize that they can form a trusting relationship with another individual, one who can accept their feelings of helplessness, neediness, and dependency, as well as their drive derivative wishes and their envy of the analyst's youthfulness (if the analyst is younger), they can be helped to cope with their problems in self-esteem. These difficulties can be traced to their genetic roots in early object-relationships, but their coming alive in interactions with the analyst gives them a sense of credence and meaning, which makes them a valuable learning experience. When older patients can think of themselves as people who can still have meaningful, or good learning experiences, this also helps them regain their capacities for regulating their self-esteem.

THE "EMPTY NEST" SYNDROME

Life Timing and How the Nest Was Emptied

Much of an older individual's response to a child growing up and leaving home depends upon the timing and manner of the child's departure. If it comes at an expected time, there will certainly be a sense of loss and of emptiness, but the disruption is not as likely to be as major as when the child's departure comes at an unexpected time or in an unexpected manner, as in the case of runaway children or children who die. The loss is not solely experienced by the mother, but is also likely to be felt by the father. The father's response has been sadly underestimated, in my experience. Many men feel a deep and genuine loss when their sons and daughters leave home and go off to school or get married.

For the woman who has primarily served as a mother, the reality of her children's growing up and going off to school or a job or a marriage, is difficult. Depending upon the relationship with the child(ren), there will be a sense of loss or of guilt (if the relationship has been a stormy one), and these emotions must be worked through in the manner of a grieving reaction. If the departure has come at an expected time, the parents will have prepared for it. They may then attempt to find other interests. The effect of the children's departure upon the relationship between the parents and with significant others, will be discussed later.

If the child's departure comes at an unexpected time, or in an unexpected manner, then there is no time to prepare for the event and it may have an overwhelming impact upon a parent. When Mrs. N, for example, lost her only son in the Vietnam war (when she was 49), and shortly thereafter lost her husband to a second heart attack, the events felt disturbingly dys-synchronous to her. Her life was thrown out of kilter and she was catapulted back to an earlier era in her existence when she had experienced a dizzying series of losses of important love objects.

She spoke of her feelings in this regard on many occasions, as when she noted: "How could I accept his [her son's] loss? I kept looking for him to walk through the door, whenever I heard a car drive up or when I heard the front doorbell ring. I found myself endlessly walking into his room and sitting down on his bed. Just sort of sitting there. Not doing anything in particular. Just kind of staring around at the bedspread and the dresser and the pictures. All of the myriad pieces of evidence of his existence. How can you ever accept that a child has died? They're still babies in your eyes, no matter how old they get. You squeezed their life out of your womb, with your own pain and tears. How can they be torn away from you like that and killed in some distant land? It's not real. It never will be!"

The depth of Mrs. N's grief, and her attempt at denial, is obvious. I am not certain that parents can ever totally acknowledge the idea of their child pre-deceasing them. It is an almost totally incomprehensible idea, one that leaves deep scars on the psyche. Such a loss must be talked about endlessly, both in and out of analysis, in order to be accepted.

In one way, Mr. W also experienced something of the "empty nest" syndrome, although long after his children's departure from the home. Even though his children had been gone from home for many years, and had been married and borne children of their own, their loss from his life was felt with an increased poignancy after the devastating series of events that brought him into analysis—his company's bankruptcy, his heart attack, and his abandonment by his wife.

From his point of view, the lack of a concrete, day-to-day impact upon the lives of the children and grandchildren made him feel less significant as a man and as a person. This is very similar to the complaints one hears from older female patients, who bemoan their lack of meaning and of identity after their children have grown up and left the "nest." They feel that their function in life is finished. Such women complain of feelings of emptiness, loss, and depression and wonder what to do with their "leftover lives." They see themselves as less attractive and less feminine (men in this position often see themselves as less aggressive and less masculine) and they may turn to drugs, such as alcohol, to escape their feelings of emptiness and despair. As noted above with Mrs. N, analyses with such people can be long and arduous, but can be brought to salutory conclusions.

Redistribution of Drive Energy

To the woman who has dedicated her life to rearing her children, their departure from the home frees a considerable amount of energy for other purposes. If this change has been long anticipated, then the redistribution of drive energy can be channeled into other avenues (hobbies, athletic interests, volunteer work, jobs, etc.) over a period of time. If the change is sudden or unexpected, particularly in parents who have not had the opportunity or the desire to develop other interests, the economy of the psyche is seriously disrupted. The parents are besieged by an upsurge of intense drive derivative wishes, of a sexual and an aggressive nature, which may overwhelm their adaptive capacities.

This difficulty with available drive energy is experienced by both parents, when their children grow up and leave home. Much of the libidinal and aggressive energy of both parents may have been previously channeled into interacting with their children. In addition to the usual libidinal and aggressive investment in children, inordinate amounts of drive energy may be tied up in certain specific (and not always pathological) parent–child relationships. When these are terminated, either expectedly or unexpectedly, this energy is released and must be expressed in other areas. If this can be done positively, as when additional libidinal energy can be invested in a mate, then object-relationships may be enhanced. If, however, these same relationships become more heavily invested with aggressive energy, they may be seriously impaired or even permanently disrupted.

If there is no available partner, as in single-parent homes, then the increased energy may be turned against the self in destructive ways, and cause great psychic pain. Mrs. N dealt with the increased increments of libidinal and aggressive energy available after the death of her son and her husband by increased alcohol consumption, withdrawal, and depression. For a variety of reasons, including conflicts over her heightened sexual desires, she was unable to turn to available objects. In gratifying herself through masturbation, she felt even guiltier and more "depraved," with a loss of self-esteem, which intensified her problem in trying to find new objects. Such difficulties are frequently seen in older patients who have grown up with values that make it difficult for them to accept that sexual and aggressive desires are normal in older people. Hence, they view themselves as moral lepers, who should be kept away, or who should keep themselves away, from others.

Changes in Object-Relationships

If the individual experiencing feelings of emptiness manages to alienate supportive love objects (or does not have supportive love objects) because of feelings of self-hatred, then a vicious circle that may ultimately lead to profound levels of despair and depression is set up. Feelings of powerlessness and helplessness contribute to a sensation that the world has slipped out of one's control, and life is chaotic. Such sensations are unpleasant and may lead to severe anxiety and to further alienation of love objects to an incapacity to find new and supportive love objects, with breakdown or suicide a possibility.

When Mrs. N came for treatment, she expressed feelings of worthlessness, because she was a "five-oh plus zero," with no husband, no children, and no social function. Her sense of herself as useless, sexually unattractive and essentially bad was intensified by virtue of her not having any significant supportive love objects in her life. This increased her identification with her alcoholic mother and led to further feelings of helplessness and despair at the idea of being trapped in an image she could neither tolerate nor respect. At such moments, patients like Mrs. N perceive their lives as essentially mirroring those of empty parents, whom they had hoped to surpass. And yet a profound longing for reunion exists with these selfsame degraded parental objects, as a means of overcoming unutterable feelings of longing and isolation. The use of drugs (alcohol, valium, cocaine, and sedatives) is a frequent sequelae in such individuals, as is depression and/or suicide. Treatment often offers the only possible avenue of interrupting the vicious circle that has been set up. In treatment, the patient recognizes the possibility of forming new object-relationships and may then be able to do so with individuals other than the therapist.

Self-esteem Regulation

As with termination of work outside the home, in the "empty nest" syndrome, those factors that contribute to the older individual's sense of themselves as being more passive, dependent, and helpless than they had perceived themselves previously, will diminish their self-esteem. The death of a child, for example, or an inharmonious departure of a child or of children from a household, will often threaten one's image of oneself as a decent person and as an individual in control of one's life. If such disruptions are accompanied by the death of or separation from an important love object, a further diminution in self-esteem may occur.

If in the course of dealing with the "empty nest" syndrome, one recognizes that one's peers are coping better with such problems than you are, then further blows to the self-esteem are incurred. This may be seen when friends whose children have also left for school decide to return to school themselves, find new jobs or volunteer positions, or undertake new and significant object-relationships. If such blows occur repeatedly, the individual may feel increasingly helpless and may withdraw. This may lead to a loss of significant friendships and to alienation from important love objects, which may then lead to more withdrawal, and a negative feedback to one's self-esteem. Unchanneled drive energy may then be increasingly turned against the self, in the absence of other avenues of discharge, and the individual may suffer increasingly from depression and from marked feelings of shame, guilt, and loss of self-esteem.

In such a setting, the individual generally will require therapy to break out of this desperate cycle. At such periods, women with strong narcissistic features (and men as well) may become more amenable to analytic intervention than they have been at other times in their lives. Such analyses are difficult, but may be very rewarding.

SUMMARY

Let me simply note that termination of one's primary occupation is a major dislocation in an individual's life, whether it is expected or unexpected. The unexpected disruptions tend to be more traumatic for most individuals, because the upsurges of instinctual drive derivatives, untoward interactions with love objects, and more radical changes in self-esteem are more intense.

11

DEALING WITH THE LOSS OF LOVE OBJECTS

One of the more important developmental issues facing the older patient is the inevitable series of object losses one faces as one grows older. Parents, mates, friends, even children may pre-decease individuals and they must learn to cope with the reality of their loss. Such deaths also call attention to one's own mortality.

If the death of a love object is expected (as the death of an old person), then grieving can be natural. If, however, the death is dyssynchronous in time with what one would normally expect, the grieving process is either aborted prematurely or is unduly prolonged.

DEATH

The most obvious example is the death of a child, as when Mrs. N's son [R] was killed in the Vietnam war. Her grief seemed never ending and inconsolable. Although such a loss is always extraordinarily painful, individuals with other object-relationships in their lives can usually resolve the loss to a considerable degree. With Mrs. N, the death of her husband, also at an unexpected time, intensified her feelings of loss and prolonged her grief response, as did the premature loss of her parents and one brother.

Repeated losses are exponential rather than additive with respect to the feelings of deprivation and sorrow older individuals experience during a grief. Although such people may appear to become inured to loss, and appear detached and almost depersonalized, underneath they are devastated, and feel helpless and hopeless. Such feelings may recall very early periods in their life, when early separations were not within their control, and appeared as absolute as death.

Feelings of helplessness tend to diminish the individual's self-esteem. This is particularly true for people who experience themselves as independent and capable of controlling their own destinies.

Many older individuals question their capacity to form new object-relationships, partly because of their diminished feelings of self-esteem. In addition, a variety of other factors (such as their overall achievements in life, relationships with their children, outside interests) play into their perceptions of themselves as people who may or may not have something to offer others, should they desire to start a new relationship. Negative self-esteem factors, such as premature job loss, a decrease in income, physical illness, the loss of a mate, may make older individuals feel so unattractive that they believe that others might wish to shun them.

The necessity to make the effort needed to form new object-relationships is often resented by some older patients. They feel that they have already paid their dues. Why should they have to extend themselves a second time in life? It hardly seems fair. Other older patients find it easier to engage themselves with new people than they had found it to be earlier in their lives. They may feel less inhibited and, because of their seeming asexuality, they can make new acquaintances, which blossom into new and important object-relationships.

A number of older patients fear that there will be no one in their lives to care for them when they get sick or to be with them at their death. I shall look at the meaning of being alone in facing death in the next chapter, but I would like to note here the intensity of the dependency needs in some older patients, which tends to parallel the range of manifestations of dependency of young children.

The feelings relevant to the subject of object losses, and the attendant grief reactions, sensations of helplessness, and issues of dependency-independency are readily manifest in the analyses of older patients. Such individuals are especially sensitive to separations in treatment, whether these separations are for weekends or for more extended holidays and vacations. I have detailed some of the more dramatic manifestations of such separation responses in the self-destructive drinking bouts of Mrs. N, in the near suicidal accident of Ms. B, and in the despair of Mr. W. Many more could have been cited. Suffice it to say, this is one of the most important features observed in the transference neuroses in such patients and it must be worked through in the transference, for the analyses to be successful. When this cannot be worked through (or it is denied or dealt with by acting out, as in the case of Mr. W) then, to that extent, the analyses are incomplete ones.

MOURNING/SEPARATION DREAMS

A fascinating feature seen in my clinical experience with older patients has to do with a particular dream phenomenon observed in five of the six patients (Mr. T, Mrs. N, Ms. B, Mr. W, and Mrs. R) discussed. Since Professor F only reported one dream during his year in treatment, I have not included him. This phenomenon involves the category of dreams reported, which is probably best described as mourning/separation. These are dreams in which the manifest content depicts either mourning for or separation from a loved one. I believe these dreams indicate the developmental importance of dealing with the subject of object losses in older patients.

Of the 609 dreams reported by Mr. T, Mrs. N, Ms. B, Mr. W, and Mrs. R, 61 (10 percent) could be described thus: 9.9 percent of Mr. T's dreams (six years of analysis), 11.3 percent of Mrs. N's (a five and one-half-year analysis), 9.1 percent of Ms. B's (four years of analysis), 8.2 percent of Mr. W's (three years of analysis), and 10.5 percent of Mrs. R's (seven years of twice-weekly psychotherapy). In all these patients, approximately 60 percent of the total number of mourning/separation dreams were reported in the last two years of their treatments (11 for Mr. T, 13 for Mrs. N, 6 for Ms. B, 4 for Mr. W, and 3 for Mrs. R, for a total of 37).

Although it is normal to anticipate the presence of dreams

involving separation anxiety in the terminal phase of analysis, I know of no precise statistics on the presence of manifest content separation dreams during this period. Thus, I have arbitrarily chosen as controls the last five patients I analyzed (in treatment with me for comparable lengths of time) who did not have any important love objects die during the course of their analyses and who completed their treatments before they reached the age of 40, well within the acceptable limits of middle, rather than old age. Of the 864 dreams reported by these five individuals over the course of their collective 27 years of analysis, only 23 (2.7 percent) depicted mourning/separation in their manifest content.

Again, of the 61 dreams reported by the older patients I have included in the mourning/separation group, 44 (72.1 percent) were dreams involving mourning for a loved one in the manifest content and 17 (27.9 percent) involved separation in the manifest content. In the younger control sample, of the 23 dreams with scenes of mourning/separation, only 3 (13 percent) involved depictions of mourning, per se; the rest involved scenes of separation.

It would be presumptuous of me to draw any far-reaching conclusions from the data presented here, but it can be safely said that my older patients reported a considerable number of dreams in which scenes of mourning for a loved one were present in the manifest content. In the younger control group, such dreams were much less frequent. Furthermore, most of the mourning dreams described by these patients occurred in the terminal phases of their psychoanalyses or psychotherapies. I have insufficient data to predict whether such dreams are characteristic of older patients, nor do I have a ready explanation for their frequent occurrence. My feeling is that they are related both to the fact that older individuals are more likely to have lost more significant objects in their lives than have younger people and to their greater proximity to their own deaths. In other words, there is a pressing need in such individuals to mourn the loss of actual love objects and the forthcoming loss of their own lives.

Something similar to this can be observed, when, during the course of an analysis, an individual loses an important love object. We may see a burst of dreams dealing with the death of the person as the mourner attempts to work through varying aspects of the loss. The death of the object has penetrated the stimulus barrier, thereby creating a type of traumatic neurosis that must be attenuated by whatever means, such as the repetition of the traumatic event in the mourner's dream life.

I would like to present here some examples of the types of dreams I have categorized as mourning/separation dreams. I might note that Mrs. N's dream of the ship draped in black (which she presented to me as a mourning dream for her father during the evaluative phase of the treatment) would be so categorized, as would Ms. B's dreams of her father's dying at a dedication ceremony for one of his buildings, or of her mother as a decaying corpse. Another of Mrs. N's dreams, which follows and which belongs in this category, occurred during the final phase of her treatment, after we had spoken of the possibility of termination.

"I had another one of my death dreams last night. This time I was with a group of women, miner's wives. There'd been an accident, a cave-in, I think, at the mines. We were all gazing down at an elevator coming up from the mineshaft with a group of bodies on it. Everyone had tears in their eyes, but they all turned toward me, as if I were supposed to be the principal mourner. I stared onto the elevator platform as it came to our level and the bodies were all covered with coal dust. Only I knew who they were right through the dust. There must have been half a dozen of them, lying there, but they all had R's [her son's] face. I began to sob and sob, and it got louder and louder and louder, until I think I woke myself up from it."

In her associations to the dream, Mrs. N said, "I think there was something about a cave-in on the news last night. No, it was the old movie, *How Green Was My Valley*, about miners. It was on TV. There was a cave-in, in it, and Maureen O'Hara loses her father, I think. And I believe that she lost her brothers, too, in earlier accidents. I'm not really sure, I was half asleep when I was watching it. Only at the end, they flashed the faces of her family on the screen, the ones who'd died or gone away and I cried like a baby when they did that. I'm a real sucker for sad films.

"I still think about R a lot. Whenever I see a reference to Vietnam in the newspapers or whenever something happens to remind me of his life. Sometimes I think that I'll never get over his death or of all the others in the family. Perhaps I hang onto all of them in my dreams, so that I won't be so lonely for them in reality.

Only I really don't feel quite so lonely anymore. I'm actually getting to like my life as it is now. Perhaps I'm finally coming to terms with all of their deaths, and with the idea that I'm going to die myself one of these days. I don't know whether you ever come to terms with that or not, but at least I'm not so scared of it now that I'm not trying to bring it on by myself. Maybe it's because we've been talking about the analysis ending and I'll be losing you, as I lost R. I don't know. It makes me sad to think that I'll be losing you, but I know it won't be the end of the world. And that's quite a change, for me to admit that!"

Another example of this variety of dream was one reported by Mrs. R late in her twice-weekly, analytically oriented psychotherapy.

"I dreamed that I went down to the mailbox to get the mail," she said. "Among the days' letters, was one that looked like an invitation to a party, only it had a thick black border all around it. My hand was trembling when I opened it up, but I was very curious about just whom the invitation was from. When I read it, it was asking me to come to a memorial service for my mother. In the dream I thought, 'but she's been dead for years!' and then I began to cry. When I awoke in the morning, the pillow was wet, so I must have actually been crying in my sleep."

In Mrs. R's associations to the dream, a number of interrelated themes emerged. The black border on the letter initially drew forth mention of the black man theme, with the concomitant idea that when her mother was out of the way, her father (the model for the black man fantasy) was more available (both emotionally and sexually). Although she had never thought that consciously at the time of her mother's death, it seemed like a very natural idea to her at the time of the dream. "Wanting my father sexually seemed a little farfetched to me," she noted, "when you first brought it up, but it doesn't seem so strange to me at all now. I think I really did want him, only he wasn't worth it. He was a very weak man."

When I inquired about the verbalization in the dream about her mother's having been dead for years, the patient noted that the anniversary of her mother's death was coming up soon. She began to cry, as she spoke of this. "Even though she never was the mother I wanted her to be," Mrs. R observed, "I still miss her a lot. Maybe it's not her so much, but the idea of being mothered, of being taken care of. I could give love to my brothers when we were children and now they can give their affection back to me. I couldn't give anything to my son when he was a baby, because of all of the black man stuff. And I can understand why he can't give me very much now. But I still feel resentful to him for not being able to. Since I've been coming to see you, I start to cry sometimes when I think of what I've never gotten from people like my parents or my own son, and never will get from them or from him. I'm still crying about it now. You won't be mad at me for being such a weak sniffling old lady, will you? I couldn't bear that, the idea of offending you. You're the only one I've got who really understands what I've lost. What I never had . . . I don't want to lose you, too."

Although there were other themes in the dream, the idea of mourning for the loss of the nurturing mother she never really had seemed the most important one. The recognition of the reasons underlying her own inability to give adequately to her own son allowed her to alleviate the guilt she felt vis-à-vis him and to establish a more reasonable relationship with him, one in which she was able to verbalize some of her feelings of resentment, as well as the long, pent-up feelings of love toward him. Her recognition of me as both the sexual father and the nurturing mother was conscious. In her associations to a terrifying dream in which she visualized my death and burial (a dream that occurred shortly after the one just described), the patient further realized that I represented both the nurturing son she did not really have and her own lost and never fully realized youth. She became extremely anxious, while associating to the dream, and the themes that emerged from it occupied her thoughts for months to come.

Although Mrs. R's acute anxiety resolved rather quickly after the dream just described, her fear of my loss remained a constant factor in the treatment. Although many sessions during the fifth year of the therapy were spent in discussing her fears of her own death, as well as the interrelated theme of the loss of my nurturing presence, the patient found it exceedingly difficult to contemplate the idea of terminating treatment. Whenever she seemed to have sufficiently worked through the issues, her anxiety would reappear, and we both recognized that it would not be feasible to set a time for stopping the sessions. We finally decided to leave the frequency of her visits up to the patient and she gradually cut down on our meetings—from twice a week to one a week and ultimately to once a month or once every six weeks. She has maintained the latter frequency for a couple of years now and she seems quite comfortable with it. She is just passing the age at which her mother died, which aroused anxiety and thoughts of reunion, but she still prefers to go on with the treatment. It is possible that she may continue with me indefinitely.

Two dreams, dealing with mourning and separation, were reported by Mr. T during the final (sixth) year of his analysis. The first is a mourning dream, the second a separation dream. Mr. T's dream of flying over Brazil and of crashing into the Amazon River (which he associated to his dead mother's name), would not be considered to be a mourning dream described in this context, as there is no direct depiction of death and mourning in the manifest content of the dream.

Shortly before his marriage to A (the blonde woman of Italian ancestry who became his third wife), Mr. T had the following dream: "My father was driving my car and I was asleep in the passenger's seat. It was raining or snowing out and the road was very wet. We were on a turnpike of some kind and the road was about to go through a tunnel in a mountain. He must have hit the brakes very hard just as we got to the tunnel, because the car went into a terrible skid and we crashed into one of the walls of the tunnel. I remember either staying asleep or losing consciousness in the dream. The next thing I knew, a rescue party came and got us out of the car, only my father was dead. I recall feeling very sad in the dream, only I wasn't able to cry."

In his associations to the dream, Mr. T said, "It's odd, dreaming about my father now. I haven't thought about him for a long time. I do feel sad though, when I think about him. I wish he were still alive, so that he could get to know A. I'm sure he'd like her. It's strange that I say that. I guess I tend to think of him growing as I have in the analysis. I see him as being a different man than he was that time with L [the Italian girl who was his childhood sweetheart]. I suppose he's come to mind again because of the wedding plans. And I guess the rain or snow that he skidded on stands for the whole spitting bit again. I think the message in the dream is that it's dangerous to be an aggressive driver or lover or husband. You can get killed, if you are. Funny how long it's taken me to come to terms with that idea. I'm not sure I'm over it yet."

His associations led to the idea of his having remained asleep during the deadly entry into the tunnel. "It's almost like pretending I'm not a man, so I don't have to risk the consequences that he did, like death. I have been thinking more about death recently. It must be because of my anxieties over the wedding. I know I'm doing the right thing, in marrying A. It's almost as if I'm making up for not having been man enough to marry L, when I was younger. It's sort of a way of reclaiming my life and my youth. But it's almost as if it's a trade-off in the dream. For me to be a man and to live, my father has to die. I think I must have always felt that way, only I never put it to myself quite that way before."

It was nearing the end of the session, but I still had some questions about the dream. I asked him what kind of car he was in, in the dream. "My car," he said, "it's a Ferrari. Oh I get it, the Italian motif again. I've always associated Italian women with both my concerns about impotency and my periods of potency. You'll get a kick out of this, doc, the car is bright red with black upholstery. Sounds pretty phallic to me."

I agreed with him about the phallic imagery and then connected the black upholstery with the color of my couch. I wondered further if his father in the dream might not also represent me and if the dream accident might be a way of articulating his fears (and wishes) about losing me, if he revealed his masculinity in the marriage to A.

"It's funny that you mention that," he noted. "I've been thinking a lot about the end of the analysis recently. It's going to be coming up pretty soon. I suppose it brings up the same concerns with you, as with my father, whether or not I can be a man without you always near me in the driver's seat. Maybe I feel there's only room for one of us in the car at a time. I'm sorry about that idea. I don't want you dead. I really care more about you than I can ever begin to say." With these thoughts, the sessions ended.

The following week, after his return from a brief business trip to another city, Mr. T reported another dream. "You know that dream I had about my father and the car last week? I had another one that reminded me of it when I was in Chicago. You and I were in a restaurant having lunch. It was as if the analysis were over and we were getting together for a pleasant meal and an amiable chat. The waiter came and brought us some champagne which you had ordered. You offered a toast of some kind to me. I'm not sure what the words were. A appeared then. I introduced her to you and she said that my face was the spitting image of yours. We both smiled when she said that and then you excused yourself to go to the bathroom, only I knew you weren't coming back. You left so quickly that I didn't have a chance to make any kind of farewell speech to you. I suddenly felt sad and scared, as if I were a little boy again, left all alone by my parents. Then A reached out for my arm and I felt a little better and the dream ended."

In his associations to the dream, the patient again spoke of our looking alike. "I guess if I'm your spitting image, I get to keep a piece of you when the analysis is over. All I have to do is look in the mirror, and I get to hang onto you. Only I think the whole spitting thing is in the dream again. If I'm an aggressive man and separate from you and marry A, then it's as if I have to get rid of you. I only send you to the bathroom in this dream, instead of killing you off as I did with my father in the last one. That's an improvement, at least. I'm not crazy about the idea of having to look like you, to still have you with me, to think of myself as a man. But it beats the hell out of being impotent."

Although there were a number of other associations to the dream, and in the days that followed important material flowed from both the dreams, what is most significant here is that they are both examples of mourning/separation dreams. Although all the dreams described in this chapter are related to the phenomenon of termination, on the one hand, there are other important elements in their genesis. One of the most prominent of these is the need to work through the deaths of or separations from important love objects in the patients' prior lives. Since older patients are more likely to have accumulated a goodly number of such losses in their lives, such dreams seem more likely to occur. With the added impetus of termination of analysis, or talk of termination, as in the case of Mrs. R, and the threat of the loss of the analyst (who serves as a transference surrogate for the lost love objects of the past), a sense of urgency is given to the need to work through this material, and hence the greater frequency of such dreams in these patients.

12
COMING TO TERMS WITH DEATH

Throughout the discussion of developmental issues facing the older individual, the issue of coming to terms with one's own impending death has been the backdrop for all the other subjects. The loss of one's powers, one's job, and one's most important objects forces the contemplation of one's own death. Yet exactly what does one have to come to terms with? What is death?

APPROXIMATIONS OF DEATH

In attempting to understand what death means to different individuals, we can only speak in terms of approximations, consistent generalizations, and idiosyncratic responses. When I speak of approximations, I am referring to specific situations that come close to death. If, for example, an individual has been in a serious accident and has been in a coma for a sustained period of time, he has "approximated" death. Just how meaningful this is, is debatable, since the individual has no particular recollection of the accident. All that remains after the trauma is the "emotional afterimage," the recognition that one has (after the fact) had an inordinately close brush with death.

Other close brushes with death, such as potentially fatal illnesses, also leave "emotional afterimages," but they do not approximate death as closely as instances in which consciousness is clouded or lost for long periods of time. Even a brief loss of consciousness approximates death, as when an individual suffers grand mal seizures or narcolepsy, undergoes electroconvulsive therapy, or is anesthetized. Sleep, too, may be so conceptualized, and disorders of sleep may often be traced to specific fears of death, especially in older individuals with chronic physical illnesses. Orgasm, as loss of self, may fit the description.

Perhaps the most devastating approximation of death involves the recognition by older individuals that their mental powers are failing. Any diminution in the mental function carries with it not only a loss in self-esteem, but also the fear of non-existence. Similarly with diseases involving the heart and, to a lesser extent, the genitals or organs of reproduction. When Mr. W had his heart attack, and before the analgesic clouded his perception of the pain, he felt that his "plane had crashed." He maintained this feeling for a long time after the episode. Patients who undergo open heart surgery may have dramatic fantasies about their scrapes with death, though few are as imaginative as the ones detailed by Bob Fosse in the film "All That Jazz."

GENERALIZATIONS ABOUT DEATH

Consistent generalizations about death refer to a series of fantasies that many people have in regard to the idea of death. A number of these have been detailed by Bibring (1966), who describes death as being conceptualized as a retaliation for destructive impulses, as the actualization of a masochistic fantasy of total surrender, or as a claustrophobic idea of being closed in on or covered over, which may be both wished for and feared. She describes death as an equivalent of castration anxiety or of fears of annihilation or of ideas of being abandoned in the dark. She further notes that it represents the loss of one's narcissistic investment in the self, as well as a loss of all one's important objects.

Ms. B's fear of having a child because she would die was the result of a fantasy that she had been responsible for her mother's death (by virtue of her having been a bad, angry child). Her own child would thus retaliate, as the dead mother's emissary, and she would be destroyed. Hence her aversion to men and to sexuality while she was still capable of bearing children. She only entered analysis after her hysterectomy had removed the possibility of childbearing.

An important determinant of Mrs. N's overindulgence in alcohol, was her wish to obliterate herself. In surrendering to liquor, her sexual and aggressive feelings would be eliminated and she would lose herself. In this manner, she would be reunited with her blob-like image of her drunken mother and undo the traumatic series of deaths that plagued her. To accomplish this, she felt that she, too, must die. On my return from a summer vacation, when we saw that Mrs. N had nearly reached the point of killing herself with her drinking, we recognized that her masochistic fantasies had almost been realized. Even her behavior with me took on a cast consistent with her fantasies. Instead of her usual feistiness, she totally and abjectly surrendered to me. In a sense, she was asking if I would concur in her wish to die, although, at the same time, she was asking me to rescue her.

Mrs. N often conceptualized many things in her life in sado-masochistic terms, particularly death. The alcohol-related deaths of mother and brother were seen as surrenders to death, as was her father's stroke while sailing. She was equivocal about her son's death in Vietnam, but she often thought of his willing the bullet to strike him. With her husband's death, which she saw as a submission to the pain that gripped his heart, it was a giving up of the ghost without a sufficient struggle. If there was no control over life and one's loved ones, then one might as well give up and accept the inevitable. Besides, in that manner, one might be reunited with all the loved dead.

Mrs. N viewed sex as surrender and orgasm as a kind of mini-death. Although this might be devoutly wished for, it was equally as devoutly feared. As the analysis progressed, and her need for masochistic fantasies lessened somewhat, her fear of death in orgasm increased until we were able to see how she connected orgasm and death in her mind.

Finally, termination of the analysis also carried with it a fantasy of inevitable surrender and the aroma of death. To lose me and my "youthful support," meant to be unprotected from a resurgence of her own self-destructiveness and a recrudescence of the wishes to surrender to the ineluctable desire for death and the reunion with lost loved ones. All this had to be analyzed as thoroughly as possible in order to ensure that she felt that she had real control over the remaining years of her life.

The conceptualization of death as a claustrophobic fantasy of being closed in on or covered over was a prevalent theme in the associations of Mrs. R. She frequently verbalized fears that she might be buried alive, and wanted her attorney to include a proviso in her will that her body would not be interred for several days. Fantasies and dreams often centered upon this topic, particularly after she read newspaper articles in which such things nearly happened.

In one such dream, she imagined herself waking from a deep sleep and still feeling very tired. She reached for the light near the bed, but found herself unable to turn it on. She then managed to stagger out of bed, to her closet. Only when she opened the closet door, she came up against a wall of earth and had the sensation of a worm crawling on her face. She awoke from this dream screaming and had to see me that day in order to assuage her fears and to assure her that her reality-testing was intact and that the terrifying vision had only been a dream.

In associating to the dream, she expressed her ongoing fears that terminating the treatment with me would result in her death. I was the light in her life. I commented that I was, more specifically, the light that she could not "turn on." The sexual connotation of my comment was apparent to her and she was able to express her anger to me over my "unwillingness" to become her sexual partner.

In proceeding further with her thoughts, she spoke of the therapy with me as having gotten her out of the closet of her sexual inhibitions, but it was all pointless without being able to find a partner to gratify her. Stepping back into the closet, which she envisioned in terms of a reunion with dead love objects, was also seen in terms of surrendering her newfound sexuality. Much as she might wish to do this, to "deaden" her desires and even her entire being, she even more intensely desired to remain alive and to feel things. Hence the presence in the dream of the phallic worm. Both sides of the conflict seemed unresolvable; hence, the anxiety.

The closet was also connected to her mother, whom we had been talking about recently. The desired closeness with her mother had never been achieved and was deeply wished for in her relationship to me in the transference. The words close and closet were seen as links to the recently expressed wishes vis-à-vis the mother, as was the association of the closet with the wish to return to her mother's womb, to start her life over again and to achieve a greater degree of gratification the second time around.

Mrs. R also feared that her recently expressed anger about her husband and his mother, who were buried side by side in a cemetery with an adjacent plot reserved for her, would lead to her demise (the feared retaliation Bibring has also spoken of in terms of fantasies about one's death). She had also recently likened her anger to me for not having gratified her sexual desires, with her anger to the husband, who never satisfied her sexually. His difficulties were seen by her as being related to his overly close ties to his mother, a woman Mrs. R had always despised. Her newly expressed wish to not be buried near her husband was seen as being too hostile, and meriting a dramatic retaliation by the dead. Her claustrophobic fantasy, in the dream, was seen as the actualization of the husband's and the mother-in-law's revenge, thereby both punishing her for her anger and gratifying, and punishing, her for the wished-for closeness to her own mother and to me, whom she wished to mother her. I might add here that the sexual desires expressed in the dream, were represented by the dirt in the closet. Although the dirt certainly depicted the ideas of death and of being buried, it also clearly portrayed the patient's feelings about her sexual desires.

It seems important to note here that many wishes and fantasies involving claustrophobic subjects not only deal with the matter of death, but also with the issue of wished-for re-birth. Mrs. R's desire to reenter the claustrum carried within it the idea of being re-born. In this second incarnation, she would receive what she had been denied in her actual life. This theme is frequently encountered in books and plays, as well as in dreams and fantasies.

The linkage between death and castration is most typically seen in patients who have suffered from life-threatening physical illnesses. The cancer victim, who has undergone mutilating surgery, or the sufferer from coronary artery disease, who has had a bypass operation, will readily attest to the connection between their near brushes with death and the perception of themselves as damaged, inadequate, and/or castrated. As noted, this is particularly poignantly seen in the case of older individuals who have suffered from some loss of their mental faculties. The perception by these individuals of their failing cognitive powers is inevitably connected with castration. In men suffering from any one of the conditions mentioned, as well as a host of others, there is a concomitant loss of self-esteem, and often depression, which may result in a loss of sexual desires and the symptom of impotency—an actual kind of castration—which intensifies the link between death and castration. The varying links between the ideas of loss of physical intactness and castration, and death and castration, must be made in the treatment to clear up the accompanying sexual performance disorder. This was very apparent in the case of Professor F, although he was unable to accept the connections between his earlier hepatitis, his beloved father-in-law's death, his impotency, and his fears of his own death, which represented the feared castration.

Fantasies of loss of one's identity are also frequently seen in connection with ideas of death. Since death obliterates one's narcissistic investment in oneself, the loss of identity is its natural sequelae. When individuals have built much of their sense of identity upon their work, their families, or their physical intactness, and one or more of these no longer are available to them, then their identities are bound to suffer. At such a time, death is seen as a natural continuation of these losses.

Mr. W's case demonstrated such connections between the idea of loss of identity and death. When the company he had devoted so much of his life to went bankrupt, he felt as if a significant aspect of himself had been eradicated. When first his physical integrity and then his marital unity were profoundly disrupted, the very core of his existence seemed threatened. He found himself entering a state of passivity and helplessness, which I have spoken of, but which was also conceptualized by him as being almost identity-less. Therefore it was logical for him to present himself to me as the fighter pilot, replete with the argot appropriate to World War II, the most successful and most concrete identity he had ever achieved. It had sustained him through the one hundred combat missions. Why shouldn't it sustain him now in his combat against a death-related non-existence?

ABANDONMENT AND SEPARATION

Another of the important equivalences in the unconscious for death is the idea of abandonment and separation. Some years ago, when I did some liaison work on a coronary care unit, I came to realize that many patients equated the idea of death with ultimate separation from their love objects. It was as if they wanted to have everyone who still counted in their lives near them, so as to impress themselves into the awareness of the others in the time that might be still allotted them. Men and women would often stare at their mates and their children as if they were trying to burn their way into them. They would often ask for familiar photographs and objects from home, so as to maintain their connections with life. Their interactions with important love objects served as a living will, in which the essence of the threatened individuals was being concretely imparted to their objects.

The threat of death intensifies the individual's recognition of all the myriad things they have not realized in their lives. The unfinished business, the failed relationships, the unrealized dreams, may all come up to haunt one at the time of one's death and may lead to intense feelings of anxiety and of separation from one's loved ones. These separation feelings may mirror early childhood feelings of actual abandonments and separations, which then may be revived with a terrifying intensity, and which may lead to the need for treatment.

An accompanying difficulty is the need to lean on one's remaining objects. Powerful dependency longings often come up in individuals who are dealing with the subject of their own deaths. When these longings can be gratified, all may be well and good, and closeness may be achieved in relationships that were never really that close before. When no close object ties exist, intense dependency needs may result in the individual's seeking out treatment to deal with their feelings of emptiness and deprivation.

The older individual frequently seeks out a young analyst or therapist, with the fantasy that the analyst's youth will protect them from death. Some patients who harbor his fantasy find it difficult to terminate their treatments (such as Mrs. R). The analyst must recognize that certain individuals may have to be supported indefinitely, since they may not be able to terminate treatment satisfactorily. As an analyst, one must also learn to deal with the envy of one's youth, which is frequently expressed covertly. It is important to work through this envy, in order to allow older patients to be better parents to their own children.

IDIOSYNCRATIC RESPONSES TO DEATH

Idiosyncratic responses to death, are unusual presentations of the idea of death. An example of this is given in a paper (Myers, 1977) on the colors black and white in dreams. In that paper, I described the case of a 51-year-old black artist I treated in psychotherapy, who frequently dreamed about being pursued by white figures. Since the patient was interested in the concept of reversals of Western values as seen in Oriental art, she consciously associated the color white with the idea of death. Another example of an idiosyncratic fantasy, although more common, is Mr. W's idea that if he remains totally passive, and doesn't overstep certain magical limits (the one-hundredth combat mission), time would stand still for him and he would not die.

A soldier's dream of a particular battlefield, where many of his buddies died, also is an idiosyncratic representation of the idea of death. However the subject is presented, its analysis is of vital importance in the treatment of the older patient.

A SUMMING UP

Although one never can totally resolve one's fears of death (and probably never should want to), one must contemplate it sufficiently to understand its consequences and its implications for the rest of one's life, as well as for the interactions with one's important objects. To do this may allow an individual to be as truly free as it is possible to be. Such freedom may make it possible to deepen old object ties and to invest in new ones, because the boundaries of life and of such ties have been explored and understood. Although I do not mean to present this as a mere existentialist exercise, there is much to be said for the concept that the recognition of one's own death lends a sweetness and an intensity to the living of one's life.

13
THE THERAPIST'S FEELINGS

A brief review of some of the major psychoanalytic articles on the subjects of transference and countertransference is in order here. I will also present data dealing with my own countertransference responses to two of the cases presented in this book.

TRANSFERENCE

One of the most penetrating insights Freud had about the subject of transference, was written early in his career (1905b) as an addenda to the Dora case. He noted that a new edition of the patient's neurosis is created during an analysis. In this new edition (the transference neurosis), all the facets of the patient's original neurotic attachment to the early objects are displaced onto the person of the analyst. Freud regarded the handling of the transference neurosis as the most difficult aspect of the analysis, but also conceptualized it as the key to the patient's believing in the connections between current behavior and the past.

In his major later papers on the subject of transference (1912, 1915, 1917), Freud dealt with the topic somewhat differently. He essentially limited his remarks about transference to the technical considerations, as when he referred to (1912) the need to interpret transference only when it prevented the free flow of associations (i.e., when it was negative or erotized). A possible factor in Freud's downplaying of the importance of transference in his later writings may have been the fact that he had no analyst of his own, although Bird (1972) notes that he did essentially utilize Fliess in this capacity. Whatever the actual reasons, in his later works, Freud (1915) shifted his emphasis from the affectual intensity of the here-and-now transference–countertransference experience between the patient and the analyst to transference as keeping the patient from remembering repressed memories.

Freud's original discussions of the transference neurosis (1905b, 1917) dealt with the transfer of symptoms onto the person of the analyst. More recent conceptualizations of the transference neurosis, such as the one by Blum (1971), focus on the broad spectrum of changes that occur under the influence of displacement of ideas and affects referable to early object representations onto the mental representation of the analyst. Thus, character neurosis is given as much importance as symptom neurosis.

More recent discussions of the general concept of transference have been influenced by the writings of such analysts as Greenacre (1968) and Greenson (1965, 1971, 1974). Greenacre traces the roots of the transference feelings toward the analyst to the early mother–child relationship and suggests that the analysand wishes the analyst to be like the omnipotent pre-oedipal mother. This may lead to a transference idealization of the analyst and to a counter-transference need, on the analyst's part, to have the patient's analysis succeed, which may predispose the analysis to failure. Mr. T's initial idealization of me, which led to a corresponding over-idealization on my part of aspects of his personality, is a good example of this, which caused some initial difficulties until I was able to understand this process.

In 1965, Greenson separated the reactions of the patient to the analyst into what he called the transference neurosis proper and the working alliance, which was defined in terms of the "reasonable feelings" the patient has for the analyst. In later papers (1971, 1972, 1974), he stressed a series of interpretive maneuvers that minimized the centrality of the transference in the analytic process. For a more detailed exposition of this subject, see my review of Greenson's collected papers (Myers, 1981).

In contrast, Gill (1979) and Gill and Hoffman (1982) emphasize the need to focus on the transference in the analysis of patients with neurosis and character neurosis. Gill refers to the patient's initial resistance to the awareness of the transference and his later resistance to the resolution of the transference. My pointing out to Mr. W that his dream of the barren lunar landscape had transference ramifications that related to my impending vacation, and that it was not simply a response to his friend's death, illustrates my attempt to deal with a resistance to the awareness of the transference. In attempting to resolve the erotized transference of Mrs. R, however, I was dealing with a resistance to the resolution of the transference. Such problems were important with all the patients described in this book, but I made little headway in this area with Professor F because of the depth of his narcissistic character structure. His need to maintain his defensive conceptualization of his grandiose self (as outlined in Kohut's 1971 discussions on narcissistic transferences) proved to be insuperable.

In an article by Blum (1973) on the concept of erotized transference, erotized transference is defined as an extreme variant of the erotic transference, characterized by vivid and irrationally erotic feelings for the analyst. It is most commonly found in patients with a history of childhood seductions or primal scene experiences and is generally accompanied by severe narcissistic vulnerability. The erotized transference generally serves as a defense against underlying feelings of hostility and may also protect the patient from becoming aware of homosexual feelings. Many of these characteristics apply to the erotized transference exhibited by Mrs. R toward me.

COUNTERTRANSFERENCE

In a review of some of the important psychoanalytic articles on the subject of countertransference, we are once again confronted with a dichotomy in Freud's writings that continues to influence theoretical writings and technical procedures. Freud initially (1910) saw countertransference as an obstructive force, which he felt should be dealt with by the analyst by a process of self-analysis. Yet almost at the same time (1912), he also verbalized the contrary notion that the analyst's unconscious could reach out toward that of the patient's and translate the patient's transmissions. In other words, the analyst's responses to the patient were then thought to be of therapeutic value.

Very little was written on the subject of countertransference during Freud's lifetime. Even the term itself was used by most classical writers in a rather narrow sense, being seen as an equivalent in the analyst of the transference in the patient (Fliess, 1953) or as the analyst's transference to the patient (Hoffer, 1956). Most writers (Fliess, 1953; Gitelson, 1952; Hoffer, 1956; Reich, 1951, 1960) of this group viewed countertransference as obstructing analysis. It was seen as arising from the analyst's neurotic conflicts and was to be dealt with by self-analysis or by further therapeutic analysis. The idea of using the feelings that arose in the analyst as a basis for understanding the patient was viewed by Reich (1960) as a substitute for true empathy, and was frowned upon.

On the other side of the controversy, analysts who were influenced by the arguments advanced by Heimann (1950) viewed countertransference in a broader way, as encompassing all the feelings the analyst experienced toward the patient. She further conceptualized the analyst's emotional responses to the patient as being of value in understanding the patient's unconscious conflicts and defenses. She did not, however, advocate communicating these responses to the patient, as A. Balint (Balint and Balint, 1939) had done.

Even more outspoken in its view, was Winnicott's (1949) brief, but controversial paper, "Hate in the Countertransference." In it, he discussed the analyst's so-called "objective countertransference," by which he meant the analyst's love and hate of his patient, presumably based on objective data emendating from the patient. Such feelings arising in the analyst were seen as being of value in both understanding the patient and in monitoring the analytic process. Winnicott saw the need to give the patient verbal feedback about the intense feelings that were being evoked in him (the analyst) and felt that such feedback served to promote the patient's maturation.

Little (1951, 1957) suggested that the patient may recognize certain real feelings in the analyst even before the analyst does and may be strongly influenced by the analyst's unconscious countertransference feelings. This view is incorporated in the approaches employed by both Searles (1958, 1978) and Langs (1976a, 1979). Little's ideas that the disturbed patient continually monitors the analyst's ability to deal with his own strong feelings is a harbinger of Bion's work (1962, 1963). Like Winnicott (1949), Little advocates the analyst's communicating these countertransference responses to disturbed patients.

Kernberg (1965), in his article on countertransference, neatly summarized the conflicting viewpoints found in this field. He refers to both classical and totalistic approaches. Adherents of the classical school (Fliess, Gitelson, Hoffer, Reich) define countertransference as the unconscious reaction of the analyst to the patient's transference, and they view countertransference as stemming from the analyst's neurotic conflicts, and thus a hindrance to analysis. Proponents of the totalistic approach define countertransference as the total emotional reaction of the analyst to the patient in the treatment situation. The analyst's responses are thus seen as being reactions to the patient's and the analyst's reality situation and to the transference milieu, as well as to the analyst's neurotic needs. To this group of writers (Heiman, Winnicott, Little, Racker), countertransference is seen as a useful therapeutic tool.

Kernberg further notes that primitive counteridentifications (as described by Fliess, 1953) may arise from partial reactivations of early ego identifications in the analyst and may pose a serious threat to the analysis by predisposing the analyst to develop certain chronic countertransference fixations. These may be manifest by reappearance of old neurotic character traits of the analyst in interactions with a particular patient; emotional discontinuance of an analysis; unrealistic total dedications to the analysis of a particular patient; and micro-paranoid attitudes toward a patient. He also notes that such problems are more likely to arise in response to patients whose conflicts are primarily concerned with elements of pregenital aggression.

I believe that all of us may go through such periods with certain patients. When Mrs. N looked depressed and defeated on my return from my summer vacation, I thought of emotionally and even literally discontinuing the analysis with her. I had similar thoughts when Ms. B took a homosexual lover. At that time, I suffered a brief emotional discontinuance of the analysis.

Several other important works remain to be mentioned in this brief survey of the literature on countertransference. One is Racker's (1968) book, *Transference and Countertransference*. Racker talks of the different identifications the analyst may experience with his patient. *Concordant identifications* are defined as those in which the analyst identifies with a segment of the psychic apparatus of the patient (ego with ego, etc.). In so doing, the analyst essentially mirrors in himself the emotion the patient is simultaneously experiencing. *Empathy* can thus be viewed as the result of a concordant identification with the patient.

Complementary identifications refer to the identifications the analyst may have with the transference objects of the patient. The analyst then is presumed to feel the emotions the patient has "put into the transference object" and the patient then re-experiences the feelings he had experienced with that particular object in the past. Racker suggests that if the analyst is made to feel that he is a bad object by the patient (by a process of projective identification), then he may feel a need to retaliate against the patient by perceiving the patient as also being bad. If the analyst recognizes this process, he will be in a position to correct the interpretive interventions.

In another article, Tower (1956) lists seven criteria to help the analyst who is suffering from some variety of countertransference difficulty. Most of these difficulties deal with handling inordinately strong affective responses the analyst may have toward the patient, as when the analyst may feel anxiety, love, or hate or may carry over affects after sessions have ended or may even dream about patients.

A number of such responses occurred in the case histories presented in this book, and I shall shortly describe some dreams I had about two of these patients. These dreams illustrate a number of the features that Tower describes. Angel (1979) also describes an instance in which a countertransference bind with a patient was resolved through the understanding of a dream. In addition, Ross and Kapp (1962) speak of translating their own countertransference responses to their patients by monitoring the visual images they were having in response to their patients' dreams.

Langs (1976a,b; 1979) suggests that countertransference expressions be kept to a minimum by the analyst, so that they do not come to dominate what he refers to as the bipersonal field. This keeps the analyst from unduly traumatizing the patient.

THE THERAPIST AND COUNTERTRANSFERENCE: RESPONSES AND DREAMS

Let me turn now to some additional details of my own countertransference responses to two of the six patients presented here. In so doing, I hope to illustrate how my own countertransference feelings affected my work with these two individuals and how I came to be aware of the difficulties I was experiencing.

I am using the word countertransference in both its broad and its narrow definitions. In the broad sense, I will describe some of my reactions from the total spectrum of my responses to the patient; in the narrow sense, I will detail some reactions that arose because of the patient's similarity in my unconscious with important love objects in my own life.

In my earlier discussion of my countertransference responses to Mr. T, I mentioned the prominent wish to rescue him. Since my own father was dying when I began the analysis of Mr. T, I believe that even my initial decision to recommend that he undergo analysis was influenced by my wish to rescue him. I might note here that my rescue fantasies vis-à-vis my own father (activated in the analysis by Mr. T's age, his specific psychological problems, etc.) resonated with the patient's own fantasies of rescuing *his* father. I feel that the reciprocal nature of our wishes contributed to the patient's strong positive transference, which was such a prominent characteristic of the analysis.

Mr. T triggered a response in me to lend him my masculine strength, so that he might live and become a more adequate man. Our joint perception of his mother as an emasculating figure, vis-à-vis both his father and himself, added to my unconscious desire to lend him my masculine power. It is possible that his subliminal awareness of my wishes in this regard may have contributed to his dreams and fantasies of younger men lending him their manly strength. Certain similarities in our familial constellations also lent substance to my identification of the patient with my father.

Although I had some rudimentary inklings of my perception of Mr. T as a father figure early in the analysis, a dream I had about him in the third month of the treatment made the matter quite clear to me.

"I was walking along the streets of a crowded Asian city with Popeye. He seemed apprehensive about not knowing his way around the place and commented upon the strangeness of the nearby signs, which were all printed in Oriental characters. For some reason, I felt no uneasiness about the place, as it seemed rather familiar to me. Then I realized that I was back in Korea again and I recognized some of the people on the street. I was about to go over and talk with one of them, when I heard the sound of bullets being fired nearby. This, too, seemed familiar and suddenly people around me began to flatten themselves against the ground in an effort to avoid being shot. Soldiers appeared and began to fire their weapons down at the bodies on the ground. I heard cries of pain and fear and I felt very angry. Then I thought of Popeye and knew that I had to get him away from the line of fire. As I gazed about me, I spied some hot red peppers drying on a nearby rooftop and I took a few of them and ate them. I felt a sudden burning surge of strength course through me and I was unconcerned about the bullets splaying all about me. At that moment, I spied Popeye lying on the ground, only he looked like Mr. T. I lifted him up onto a nearby rooftop, out of the path of the gunfire. With that I breathed a sigh of relief, though I awoke shortly thereafter, feeling somewhat anxious."

There are many associations I might offer to this dream, but I shall only list a few of the more pertinent ones. Popeye immediately struck me as being a reference to my father, not only for the obvious verbal reference to "pop," but also because of a pleasant childhood memory I had about my father, involving his showing me 8-millimeter movies, one a Popeye comedy. The juxtaposition of Mr. T with Popeye in the dream illustrates my connection of the two men in my mind. In addition, there is the obvious wish that both needed to be saved and that I am the one who can do it. Popeye—Mr. T is on unfamiliar ground, the analysis, where I know my way around.

The city is Seoul, a place I knew well from my military service there, and the scene of the soldiers firing into the crowd, was taken from the revolution in which Syngman Rhee was deposed, which I had lived through. Bad as Rhee was, I saw his wife as being worse, which was consistent with the picture I had at that time of Mr. T's familial constellation (and with some residual distortions I harbored at that time about my own family).

As a consequence of the revolution in Korea, I lost contact with a woman I had been close to, an obvious identification with Mr. T's loss of L (his childhood and adolescent girlfriend). My identification with him becomes even clearer, when I become a kind of Popeye figure myself, in the process of eating the red peppers. These fiery red vegetables are the obvious counterpart of the usual green spinach from a can.

I could go on about the dream, but I will leave it at this point. Suffice it to say, it seems obvious that my countertransference wish to rescue Mr. T is quite patently represented in it. My recognition of the archaic nature of the wish and of the childhood conflicts it was meant to undo, led to the anxiety that awakened me from the dream.

Following the analysis of this dream, I was also able to recognize certain negative feelings I had harbored toward the patient, especially when he failed to be the idealized father figure I had wanted him to be. I could then see that my early tendency to dilute early transference interpretations to him, so as to avoid further narcissistic mortification, was based on my own need to minimize my hostility to him generated by my perception of him as a devalued father figure.

In the period right after my father's death, I also noted pangs of separation anxiety in myself whenever the patient was away on an unexpected business trip. By virtue of my working through the important countertransference responses that arose during the analysis of Mr. T, I was able to work through many important pieces of my mourning response for my own father. In this sense, the analysis had invaluable consequences for both of us.

Moving on now to Mrs. N, let me note that my initial response to her was positive. She was an intelligent woman and was still quite attractive physically, in spite of her depression and her overindulgence in alcohol. She also bore something of a superficial resemblance to my former analyst, an older woman whose background resembled hers. Although this enhanced my attraction to her in one way, in another, certain unresolved negative transference feelings toward my former analyst were also displaced by me onto the patient. Her initial presentation as a competitive, castrating woman also made me feel irritated with her and wish to strike back at her. These feelings also had roots in certain unresolved feelings for my former analyst. I once more became aware of this countertransference attitude when I dreamed about the patient early in the course of her treatment.

"In the dream, the patient and I were dressed in fencing clothes. Each of us held foils and were moving down the mat toward each other. Then we engaged our foils and began to duel. For a number of moments, she parried my every thrust and I felt quite frustrated. Then she thrust at me with her foil and I parried and immediately riposted. With that movement, I scored a touché and she fell down on the mat. I stood over her with my foil poised, and she gazed up at me with an imploring look on her face. I felt a sudden surge of warmth for her and put my foil down and offered her my hand to help her up."

The sexual symbolism in the dream is fairly obvious. But in associating to the dream, I thought a good deal about the irritation and the fear engendered in me by Mrs. N's competitiveness and her phallic envy. Obviously it aroused some castration anxiety in me and I retaliated by besting her in the fencing match (a sport I had been quite good at, as opposed to tennis, which would have been her game). Mrs. N also reminded me of a woman I had been involved with during the period in my life when fencing had been important to me. This woman was an excellent fencer, but she lacked the competitiveness and phallic envy that so characterized the patient's interactions toward men. The obvious wish in the dream was that Mrs. N would become modified, so as to be more like my former girlfriend. The woman's name was similar to that of my former analyst, hence I was able to recognize this as being important in terms of my feelings to the patient. The dream also enabled me to lay to rest a certain residual irritation I had felt toward my former analyst after the termination of my analysis. The childhood roots of the dream were also apparent to me, in my representation of the patient as a fallen, aphallic mother figure whom I could then feel warmth and love toward, without any risk of being emasculated.

With the analysis of the dream, I was able to understand my own attitude toward the patient more adequately. In addition, I could more clearly comprehend her own need to defensively adopt the stance of the phallic woman, in order to deal with her sense of herself as castrated, following the loss of all the significant male figures in her life.

When her drinking was at its zenith, and I feared for the viability of the analysis, I was disappointed with and irritable toward the patient. By self-analysis, I was able to relate this feeling further to certain disappointments with mothering figures in my own life, such as my own mother and my female analyst. For brief intervals during this period of self-analysis, I became detached from the patient—the emotional discontinuation of the analysis that Kernberg (1965) speaks of in his paper on countertransference. My detachment likely contributed to the patient's perception of me at such times as being distant and unreachable, as in the dream in which she screams out and I do not respond to her. Fortunately, I sufficiently resolved the difficulties within myself and the analysis proceeded successfully.

In my countertransference responses to Ms. B, both protective and sadistic impulses were elicited, over and above the usual amount elicited by masochistic characters. I think this may have been related to her long-standing virginity and her sexual innocence. She seemed a battered child to me, or perhaps a naif, clearly someone who needed help. To relate to her in this mode was to set myself up for her sadistic attacks and to recoil from them (in other words, to abandon her temporarily). Her rage was difficult to withstand, but its most profound statement came through her intuiting my investment in her achieving heterosexuality. Once she saw this, she unconsciously knew how to strike at me. Certainly her relationship with Ellen had many other determinants besides this, but my initial response to her announcement of it was as if this was the only operant cause. The depth of her happiness with Ellen surprised me. It taught me to be much less judgmental about the relationships of lesbian women and gay men.

My own responses to Mr. W were painful for me to handle at first, related as they were to the final illness of my brother, but they had been apparent to me from the beginning of the treatment. This made it easier for me to see them and to deal with them, hence they never caused any major interference of my analytic stance. His jealousy and envy of my youth were never that bitter and vindictive, hence I had no real problem dealing with these areas.

I was disappointed that he decided to terminate treatment, but I felt that I had done all that I could have done to help him to stay, so I did not feel guilty about having missed any area I might have interpreted to him. Basically, however, I felt that the treatment was a rewarding one for the two of us and I had no regrets that I had recommended analysis as the treatment of choice.

My countertransference responses to Mrs. R were intense, since the patient's age and seductiveness reactivated within me my own oedipal strivings. The fantasies thus elicited led to my initial reluctance to interpret the obvious oedipal data she was presenting and to deal with the transference feelings she was expressing toward me. Only through a process of self-analysis, was I able to surmount this initial difficulty. In so doing, I was able to understand certain feelings toward my own analyst to a greater degree than I had during my own training analysis.

Finally, let me note the countertransference responses I felt toward Professor F. From my description of the case, it is apparent that I experienced him as difficult to work with. Although narcissistic personality disorders are notorious for causing negative countertransference responses in analysts and therapists alike, I have had a fair modicum of success with such patients in the past. I believe that part of my difficulty with Professor F stemmed from my wish to repeat my prior therapeutic success with Mr. T. Another way of stating this would be to say that I desired to resurrect my lost father and the patient thwarted my ability to realize this important fantasy. As a result, I felt quite angry toward him and had difficulty forcing myself to confront the reasons for this feeling. When I did not confront these reasons, I found myself acting out my identifications with his unconscious needs, rather than attempting to analyze them.

What this case once more illustrates is the vital importance of monitoring one's own countertransference responses toward one's patients. This seems to me to be of especial importance in dealing with older patients, who may evoke responses that are displacements of prominent feelings toward, or fantasies about, one's parents or one's own analyst. These countertransferences are hardly insurmountable. In working through them, the analyst has an important opportunity for self-analysis and a chance to come to terms with certain unresolved aspects of his own training analysis. This latter feature is especially likely to be true when the patient is older than the analyst.

14
THE USEFULNESS OF DYNAMIC THERAPY WITH THE OLDER PATIENT

Here I would like to summarize some of the findings detailed earlier in the book. The first and foremost conclusion that can be derived from a reading of the clinical data presented is that psychoanalysis of older patients (over 50) is both feasible and useful. The four analyses proper described in the book had salutory results, as did one of the two psychoanalytic psychotherapies. Although not all the analyses went as far as I might have wished them to, similar statements could be made regarding analyses of patients in any age group. In essence, Freud's dicta against analyzing people over the age of 50, because of their presumed ineducability and their inelasticity, was unwarranted, unwise, and inaccurate.

From the material presented, it is clear that the analyses of older patients do not materially differ from those of younger patients. Certain issues, such as the increasing frequency of object loss, the feelings attendant upon the termination of work, and the coming to terms with one's own death may stand out, but the analyses themselves are not greatly altered by the urgency of these issues. Regardless of the age of the individual, if the patient is not suffering from significant organic brain disease, lost memories may be recovered and longstanding symptomatic characterological disturbances may be modified.

It is also quite clear that the older patient can form the same intensity of transference relationships as can patients of any age group. One need only turn to the erotized transference of Mrs. R, who entered psychotherapy at the age of 71, to prove this point. Oedipal issues are also as prominent in this population as they are in any other age group. These findings contrast with those reported by Sandler (1978) in an analysis she performed on an older patient, but my findings are consistent throughout the cases reported in this book and are compatible with my findings with other older patients I have worked with.

ASSESSMENT OF ANALYZABILITY

In assessing analyzability in this age group, the usual factors that influence analyzability in any age group pertain. In addition, certain factors specifically related to the age of these patients determines whether they are treatable or not. In this regard, let me single out the so-called "last chance" idea cited by King (1980). What this amounts to is that a tremendous impetus may be given to the motivation for treatment by virtue of these individuals recognition that this may be their last opportunity to change their lives. This seems to be even more prominent when these patients are either nearing the age at which a parent may have died or an age at which some other negative and limiting factor became apparent in the life of a parent or other close love object.

Analyzability in older people is also influenced by whether or not they have come to terms with their own achievements and themselves, as well as with their love objects. Those individuals who are able to accept the limitations of their own lives, and their love objects, seem to be more amenable to analysis or analytic psychotherapy than those who have not. The increment of envy possessed by patients in this age group is important here. Those who are extremely envious of the youth of others (children, subordinates, analysts) are less likely to be helped significantly. They will either unconsciously attempt to destroy the treatment in order to prove the impotence of the analyst (as Professor F did with me), and thus diminish their envy, or the invidious comparisons they draw between themselves and their analysts will depress them too much. In either event, too high a titer of envy in a patient is likely to predispose the treatment to failure.

Losses of Aspects of the Self

In dealing with the older patient, it is important to understand certain developmental issues. When we consider, for example, the concept of loss of various aspects of the self in the aging process, certain features stand out. Not only does a diminution or a loss of one's athletic ability make one feel older, but it may also mean the weakening of an important object tie (even if the actual object that tied one to the particular sport has died). Similarly with losses of (or decreases in) sensory acuity (vision, hearing). These may lead to feelings of sensory deprivation, to a diminishment in self-esteem, and to ideas of being "freakish," which may be unconsciously equated to castration. To lose one's reproductive capacity, or to become less potent, also diminishes self-esteem and leads to feelings of being castrated and "old." When we add in the idea of the loss of sexual attractiveness, the potential loss of the capacity to find new partners for sexual interactions is very threatening to certain individuals, especially narcissistic ones.

Patients whose intellectual or cognitive functions have changed conceive of themselves as deteriorating and as unattractive to others. They may become irritable and defensive, which may further alienate them from real or potential love objects and lead to an ever-increasing sense of isolation and loneliness. Because the intellect is phallicized in so many individuals, changes (which may be accompanied by feelings of depression) in intellectual and cognitive functioning may make such people feel "castrated."

Physical illness in the older patient also has emotional aspects. When prized organs, such as the heart and the brain, are involved, the patient generally experiences an intense castration anxiety. This anxiety tends to affect sexual functioning, which may lead to marked interferences in object-relationships, as occurred in the case of Mr. W.

Thus, all aspects of losses of the self can be seen as leading to losses in self-esteem and to alienation from real or potential love objects. Successful analytic treatment in this age group must lead to a greater degree of acceptance of physical and mental limitations.

The idea of termination of work in the older individual, even under the best of circumstances, is apt to be a major dislocation. Much of the response to such a change, however, depends on whether the change is unexpected. If it is, then problems are more likely.

Stopping Work

When one leaves a job voluntarily, one is left with a sensation of control over one's life, whereas being forced out of a job unexpectedly and involuntarily leaves one feeling helpless. Stopping a job also leads to a need to re-direct the libidinal and aggressive drive energy that has been channeled into work. Again, if the work stoppage is unexpected, the drive re-direction may be interfered with by dysphoric affects, such as anxiety and depression, which may also abet the feeling of being helpless and of one's life being out of control.

And if individuals have no sympathetic and supportive love objects available to them (as in the case of Mrs. R), a sudden upsurge in drive energy (as when her libidinal feelings became increasingly available to her) may lead to the feeling of being besieged by one's drives. Masturbation may become almost compulsive and frenzied, with an accompanying sense of profound shame and guilt, until the treatment is able to mitigate these affects. Such individuals often re-experience the adolescent sense of being a passive victim of overwhelming drives, which are seen as being "unseemly" for individuals of their age.

Individuals who have stopped working (especially if this was not of their own choice) may suffer from feelings of loss of self-esteem or even of self-hatred. These may become so intense that they may even push away sympathetic and supportive love objects, which further increases their sense of self-hatred and isolation. For some people, such as Mr. W, the acknowledgment of dependency needs is anathema and a sign of weakness, which is seen as being equivalent to castration. This leads to a denial of legitimate dependency gratifications and to an alienation from love objects.

Changes in friendships, as a result of social and financial pressures after job stoppage, also affect positive object-relationships in older individuals. All these factors can lead to sensations of passivity and helplessness and to feelings of frustration and anger (often turned against the self), which play havoc with the individual's self-esteem.

The "Empty Nest" Syndrome

Many of the features described as being of importance in stopping a job, also pertain to the so-called "empty nest" syndrome. The departure of children is most disruptive when the circumstances are either very negative (as in a parent–child relationship clouded by constant conflict) or totally dys-synchronous (as when a child dies). Men, as well as women, suffer from the effects of this syndrome and an appropriate period of grieving is needed for both parents.

Parents who suffer intensely from the "empty nest" syndrome speak of dysphoric affects (anxiety and depression) and complain of feelings of emptiness, loss, and concern about what to do with their "leftover lives." They see themselves as being less attractive, or less feminine or masculine, and they may turn to drugs or alcohol.

Needless to say, much drive energy is tied up in the object-relationships parents have with their children. When these are interrupted or terminated—by children moving out of the home or dying—this energy becomes available for other uses. Without sympathetic love objects or significant relationships or avocations into which to channel this energy, it may be perceived of as overwhelming and may lead to dysphoric affects.

Mourning/Separation Dreams

When one turns from the normal separations faced by most parents as their children leave the home to the plethora of object losses the older individual must deal with as the years go by, we come face to face with one of the most poignant problems for older people. In this setting, I have observed an interesting phenomenon that occurred in five of my six patients. The phenomenon has to do with a special category of dreams reported by these five individuals, a category best described as mourning/separation dreams.

Approximately 10 percent of the dreams reported by these five patients could be included in this category, with nearly six of ten of these dreams being reported by these individuals in the last two years of treatment. In comparing this finding with the dreams of patients who completed their analyses by the age of 40, less then 3 percent of their dreams could be so categorized. I see this as being related to the greater actual number of lost love objects suffered by the older age group and to their greater proximity to their own deaths. In other words, such individuals must mourn not only for actual love objects lost in the past, but also for the forthcoming loss of their own selves.

Death

In dealing with the subject of death itself, the best we can do is to look at what I would refer to as close approximations of death, consistent generalizations about death, and idiosyncratic responses to death. By approximations, I mean those situations that come closest to death, such as coma, or other inordinately close brushes with death an individual may experience.

Consistent generalizations about death refers to the fantasies many people have with respect to the idea of death. Bibring's (1966) exposition of death as being viewed as a retaliation for one's destructive impulses, as the actualization of a masochistic fantasy of total surrender, or as a claustrophobic idea of being covered over are important here. In addition, fear of death may be seen as the equivalent of castration anxiety, fears of annihilation, or anxieties about being abandoned. Idiosyncratic responses, in single individuals, refer to their own peculiar conceptualizations of and fantasies about death. The idea of remaining totally passive, in order to avoid the passage of time and of getting older and dying (as expressed by Mr. W), is an example of such a fantasy.

Although one never overcomes one's fear of death, one may come to terms with its implications and consequences. To truly do so, allows for a freedom that may deepen old object ties and allow new ones to be formed. This happens because the boundaries of life and of object ties have been explored and understood.

COUNTERTRANSFERENCE

Countertransference responses as experienced by the analyst in dealing with the older patient are also important. These may be countertransference responses, in the narrow sense, related to love objects from one's own past life (parents or one's own analyst) or they may be countertransference responses in the broader sense, involving any and all of one's responses to the patient.

The specific nature of such countertransference responses depends upon the age of the analyst vis-à-vis the age of the patient. If the analyst is significantly younger, the analyst must learn to deal with the sexuality of these older patients and their envy of the analyst's youth (what might be called the Dracula syndrome, wherein an older patient attempts to suck up the youth of the younger analyst so as not to recognize the aging processes and the imminence of death). In dealing with such dramatic transference and countertransference manifestations, the analyst can perform a significant piece of self-analysis, which, as a side effect, helps resolve long-standing neurotic conflicts involving the analyst's parents and training analyst.

REFERENCES

Abraham, K. (1919). The applicability of psycho-analytic treatment to patients at an advanced age. In *Selected Papers*, pp. 312–317. New York: Basic Books, 1953.

Alexander, F. (1944). The indications for psychoanalytic therapy. *Bulletin of the New York Academy of Medicine, Second Series* 20(6):319–332.

Angel, E. (1979). The resolution of a countertransference through a dream of the analyst. *The Psychoanalytic Review* 66:9–17.

American Psychoanalytic Association (1982). Discussion group on: Psychoanalytic contributions to the psychology of aging, including a case report of the psychoanalysis of an elderly patient. Co-chairmen M. A. Berezin and W. Tarnower, 12/15/82.

American Psychoanalytic Association (1982). Panel on: The psychoanalysis of the older patient. Chaired by M. A. Berezin, 12/19/82.

APA Task Force on the 1981 White House Conference on Aging (1981). Abstracted as: APA contends elderly "consistently underserved." In *Psychiatric News*, October 16, 1981, p. 10ff.

Balint, A. and Balint, M. (1939). On transference and countertransference. *International Journal of Psycho-Analysis* 20:223–230.

Berezin, M. A. (1963). Some intrapsychic aspects of aging. In *Normal Psychology of the Aging Process*, ed. N. E. Zinberg and I. Kaufman, pp. 93–117. New York: International Universities Press, Inc.

——— (1965). Introduction. In *Geriatric Psychiatry. Grief, Loss, and Emotional Disorders in the Aging Process*, ed. M. A. Berezin and S. H. Cath, pp. 13–20. New York: International Universities Press, Inc.

———, Birren, J. E., Cath, S. H., Levin, S., Michaels, J. J. and Zetzel, E. R. (1965). Discussion. In *Geriatric Psychiatry. Grief, Loss, and Emotional Disorders in the Aging Process,* ed. M. A. Berezin and S. H. Cath, pp. 120–142. New York: International Universities Press, Inc.

Bibring, G. L. (1966). Old age: Its liabilities and its assets. A psychobiological discourse. In *Psychoanalysis, a General Psychology,* ed. R. Loewenstein, pp. 253–271. New York: International Universities Press, Inc.

Bion, W. (1962). *Learning from Experience.* New York: Basic Books.

——— (1963). *Elements of Psychoanalysis.* New York: Basic Books.

Bird, B. (1972). Notes on transference: universal phenomenon and hardest part of analysis. *Journal of the American Psychoanalytic Association* 20:267–301.

Blum, H. P. (1971). On the conception and development of the transference neurosis. *Journal of the American Psychoanalytic Association* 19:41–53.

——— (1973). The concept of erotized transference. *Journal of the American Psychoanalytic Association* 21:61–76.

Bradlow, P. (1981). Personal communication.

Busse, E. W. (1965). Research on aging: some methods and findings. In *Geriatric Psychiatry. Grief, Loss, and Emotional Disorders in the Aging Process,* ed. M. A. Berezin and S. H. Cath, pp. 73–93. New York: International Universities Press, Inc.

Cath, S. H. (1965). Some dynamics of middle and later years: A study in depletion and restitution. In *Geriatric Psychiatry. Grief, Loss, and Emotional Disorders in the Aging Process,* ed. M. A. Berezin and S. H. Cath, pp. 21–72. New York: International Universities Press, Inc.

Cohler, B. J. and Milke, N. E. (1983). NIMH holds First Conference on Aging. Psychoanalytic perspective featured. Newsletter, The American Psychoanalytic Association, April 1983, pp. 8–9.

Committee on Psychoanalytic Practice of the American Psychoanalytic Association (1980). Co-chairmen D. Jaffe and D. Shapiro, p. 59.

Erikson, E. H. (1959). *Identity and the Life Cycle. Psychological Issues Monograph,* Vol. 1, pp. 1–171. New York: International Universities Press, Inc.

Fliess, R. (1953). Counter-transference and counter-identification. *Journal of the American Psychoanalytic Association* 1:268–284.

Freud, S. (1898). Sexuality in the aetiology of the neuroses. *Standard Edition* 3:261–285.

——— (1904). Freud's psycho-analytic procedure. *Standard Edition* 7:249–254.
——— (1905a). On psycho-therapy. *Standard Edition* 7:257–268.
——— (1905b). Fragment of an analysis of a case of hysteria. *Standard Edition* 7:3–122.
——— (1910). The future prospects of psycho-analytic therapy. *Standard Edition* 11:139–152.
——— (1912). Recommendations for physicians practising psychoanalysis. *Standard Edition* 12:109–120.
——— (1915). Observations on transference love. *Standard Edition* 12:157–173.
——— (1917). Introductory lectures on psycho-analysis. *Standard Edition* 16:431–447.
Giambra, L. N. (1977). Daydreaming about the past: the time setting of spontaneous thought intrusions. *Gerontologist* 17:35–38.
Gill, M. M. (1979). The analysis of the transference. *Journal of the American Psychoanalytic Association.* Suppl. 27:263–288.
——— and Hoffman, I. Z. (1982). *Analysis of Transference.* Vols. 1 and 2. New York: International Universities Press, Inc.
Gitelson, M. (1952). The emotional position of the analyst in the psychoanalytic situation. *International Journal of Psycho-Analysis* 33:1–10.
——— (1965). A transference reaction in a sixty-six year old woman. In *Geriatric Psychiatry. Grief, Loss, and Emotional Disorders in the Aging Process.* ed. M. A. Berezin and S. H. Cath, pp. 160–186. New York: International Universities Press, Inc.
Goldfarb, A. I. (1963). A psychosocial and sociophysiological approach to aging. In *Normal Psychology of the Aging Process*, ed. N. E. Zinberg and I. Kaufman, pp. 72–92. New York: International Universities Press, Inc.
Greenacre, P. (1968). Problems of overidealization of the analyst and the analysis. *Psychoanalytic Study of the Child* 21:193–212.
Greenson, R. R. (1965). The working alliance and the transference neurosis. *Psychoanalytic Quarterly* 34:155–181.
——— (1971). The "real" relationship between the patient and the psychoanalyst. In *The Unconscious Today: Essays in Honor of Max Schur*, ed. M. Kanzer, pp. 213–232. New York: International Universities Press, Inc.
——— (1972). Beyond transference and interpretation. *International Journal of Psycho-Analysis* 53:213–217.
——— (1974). Loving, hating and indifference toward the patient. *International Review of Psycho-Analysis* 1:259–266.

Grotjahn, M. (1940). Psychoanalytic investigation of a seventy-one year old man with senile dementia. *Psychoanalytic Quarterly* 9:80–97.
—— (1951). Some analytic observations about the process of growing old. *Psychoanalysis and the Social Sciences* 3:301–312.
—— (1955). Analytic psychotherapy with the elderly. *The Psychoanalytic Review* 42:419–427.
Heimann, P. (1950). On countertransference. *International Journal of Psycho-Analysis* 31:81–84.
Hoffer, W. (1956). Transference and transference neurosis. *International Journal of Psycho-Analysis* 37:377–379.
Hurn, H. T. (1969). Synergic relations between the processes of fatherhood and psychoanalysis. *Journal of the American Psychoanalytic Association* 17:437–451.
Jacques, E. (1970). *Work, Creativity, and Social Justice.* New York: International Universities Press, Inc.
Kaufman, M. R. (1937). Psychoanalysis in late-life depression. *Psychoanalytic Quarterly* 6:308–335.
Kaufman, I. (1963). Psychodynamic considerations in normal aging. In *Normal Psychology of the Aging Process,* ed. N. E. Zinberg and I. Kaufman, pp. 118–124. New York: International Universities Press, Inc.
Kernberg, O. F. (1965). Notes on countertransference. *Journal of the American Psychoanalytic Association* 13:38–56.
—— (1980). *Internal World and External Reality. Object Relations Theory Applied.* New York: Jason Aronson, Inc.
King, P. (1980). The life cycle as indicated by the nature of the transference in the psychoanalysis of the middle-aged and the elderly. *International Journal of Psycho-Analysis* 61:153–160.
Klein, M. (1963). *Our Adult World.* New York: Basic Books.
Kohut, H. (1971). *The Analysis of the Self.* New York: International Universities Press, Inc.
Langs, R. J. (1976a). *The Bipersonal Field.* New York: Jason Aronson, Inc.
—— (1976b). *The Therapeutic Interaction,* Vols. 1 and 2. New York: Jason Aronson, Inc.
—— (1979). *The Therapeutic Environment.* New York: Jason Aronson, Inc.
Levin, S. (1965a). Some comments on the distribution of narcissistic and object libido in the aged. *International Journal of Psycho-Analysis* 46:200–208.
—— (1965b). Depression in the aged. In *Geriatric Psychiatry. Grief, Loss, and Emotional Disorders in the Aging Process,* ed. M. A. Berezin

and S. H. Cath, pp. 203–225. New York: International Universities Press, Inc.

Linden, M. E. (1963). Regression and recession in the psychoses of the aging. In *Normal Psychology of the Aging Process*, eds. N. E. Zinberg and I. Kaufman, pp. 125–142. New York: International Universities Press, Inc.

Little, M. (1951). Countertransference and the patient's response to it. *International Journal of Psycho-Analysis* 32:32–40.

────── (1957). The analyst's response to his patient's needs. *International Journal of Psycho-Analysis* 38:240–254.

McMahon, A. W. and Rhudick, P. J. (1967). Reminiscing in the aged: An adaptational response. In *Psychodynamic Studies on Aging. Creativity, Reminiscing, and Dying,* ed. S. Levin and R. J. Kahana, pp. 64–78. New York: International Universities Press, Inc.

Meerloo, J. A. M. (1953). Contribution of psychoanalysis to the problems of the aged. *Psychoanalysis and Social Work*, ed. M. Heimann. New York: International Universities Press, Inc.

────── (1955). Transference and resistance in geriatric psychotherapy. *The Psychoanalytic Review* 42:72–82.

Myers, W. A. (1976). Imaginary companions, fantasy twins, mirror dreams, and depersonalization. *Psychoanalytic Quarterly* 45:503–524.

────── (1977). The significance of the colors black and white in the dreams of black and white patients. *Journal of the American Psychoanalytic Association* 25:163–181.

────── (1979). Imaginary companions in childhood and adult creativity. *Psychoanalytic Quarterly* 48:292–307.

────── (1980). The psychodynamics of a beating fantasy. *International Journal of Psychoanalytic Psychotherapy* 8:623–648.

────── (1981). Review of: *Explorations in Psychoanalysis by R. R. Greenson.* New York: International Universities Press, Inc. In *Psychoanalytic Quarterly* 50:272–275.

Neugarten, B. L. (1970). Dynamics of transition of middle age to old age. Adaptation and the life cycle. *Journal of Geriatric Psychiatry* 4:71–87.

Racker, H. (1968). *Transference and Countertransference.* New York: International Universities Press, Inc.

Reich, A. (1951). On countertransference. *International Journal of Psycho-Analysis* 32:25–31.

────── (1960). Further remarks on countertransference. *International Journal of Psycho-Analysis* 41:389–395.

Ross, D. W. and Kapp, F. T. (1962). A technique for self-analysis of countertransference. *Journal of the American Psychoanalytic Association* 10:643–657.

Sandler, A. M. (1978). Psychoanalysis in later life. Problems in the psychoanalysis of an aging narcissistic patient. *Journal of Geriatric Psychiatry* 11:5-36.

Searles, H. (1958). The schizophrenic's vulnerability to the therapist's unconscious processes. *Journal of Nervous and Mental Disease* 127:247-262.

——— (1978). Psychoanalytic therapy with the borderline adult. In *New Perspectives on Psychotherapy with the Borderline Adult,* ed. J. Masterson. New York: Brunner/Mazel.

Segal, H. (1958). Fear of death. Notes on the analysis of an old man. *International Journal of Psycho-Analysis* 39:178-181.

Shainess, N. (1979). Analyzability and capacity for change in middle life. *Journal of the American Academy of Psychoanalysis* 7:385-403.

Strachey, J. (1934). The nature of the therapeutic action of psychoanalysis. *International Journal of Psycho-Analysis* 15:127-159.

Tower, L. E. (1956). Countertransference. *Journal of the American Psychoanalytic Association* 4:224-255.

Winnicott, D. S. (1949). Hate in the countertransference. *International Journal of Psycho-Analysis* 30:69-74.

Wolff, K. (1971). Individual psychotherapy with geriatric patients. *Psychosomatics,* 12:89-93.

Zinberg, N. E. and Kaufman, I. (1963). Cultural and personality factors associated with aging: an introduction. In *Normal Psychology of the Aging Process,* ed. N. E. Zinberg and I. Kaufman, pp. 17-71. New York: International Universities Press, Inc.

Index

Abraham, K., 2, 169
Adolescence
  biological and sexual similarity
    to old age, 11
Alcohol utilization by older
    individuals, 41–67, 174,
    200–202, 217
Alexander, F., 3, 170
Analyzability of the older patient.
    See also Treatability of older
    patient, evaluation of,
    169–180
  accessibility of unconscious
    material (dreams and
    fantasies), 23, 49–51, 116–117,
    155, 167, 173–174, 177–179
  continuing capacity for pleasure,
    24, 52, 81, 167, 173–174, 176
  degree of masochism, 52, 58, 66,
    80, 175
  degree of passivity, 51, 115–116,
    174, 176
  familial constellation of patient,
    173, 175, 178
  history of depersonalization, 76,
    80, 175
  increased motivation due to aging,
    11, 23–24, 66–67, 170–173,
    175, 177–178, 180
  intensity of envy possessed by
    patient, 4–5, 9, 12–13,
    170–171, 174
  literature on evaluation of, x–xi,
    1–13
  narcissistic personality structure,
    13, 161, 166–167, 179
  potential for formation of
    transference neurosis, 23, 51,
    114, 155–156, 159, 173–174,
    177, 179

Analyzability of the older patient (*continued*)
  prior physical illness, 157, 177
  quality of object-relationships, 2, 5–10, 12–13, 23, 39, 51–52, 79–81, 106, 119, 143, 155, 159, 167, 175, 177–179
  therapist's rescue fantasies, 24, 29, 115, 159
American Psychoanalytic Association, discussion group and panel, ix
Angel, E., 228
APA Task Force on the 1981 White House Conference on Aging, ix

Balint, A., and Balint, M., 226
Berezin, M. A., 7
Bibring, G. L., 216, 242
Bion, W., 227
Bird, B., 224
Blum, H. P., 224–225
Boston Society for Gerontological Psychiatry, 6, 8
Bradlow, P., 180
Busse, E. W., 7

Case of Ms. B, 69–106
  countertransference issues, 87–93, 99, 102
  dreams, 83–85, 95, 105
  factors affecting analyzability, 79–83, 106
  fears of death, 84, 100
  sexuality, 78–79, 95–98, 101–102, 106
  termination, 100, 104
  transference issues, 83, 85–93, 98, 103–104
Case of Professor F, 157–167
  countertransference issues, 161, 163
  factors affecting analyzability, 159–160, 162, 166–167
  fears of death, 164–166
  sexuality, 158, 161–162
  transference issues, 162
Case of Mrs. N, 41–67
  countertransference issues, 52, 54–55, 58
  dreams, 49–51, 57–58
  factors affecting analyzability, 51–52, 66–67
  fears of death, 65
  free association, 51
  narcissistic issues, 52
  sexuality, 59–61, 63–64
  termination, 65
  transference issues, 50–51, 53–56, 58–61, 64, 67
Case of Mrs. R, 145–156
  countertransference issues, 148, 151
  dreams, 152–153, 210–211, 218–219
  factors affecting analyzability, 155–156
  fears of death, 218–219
  free association, 147–149, 155
  sexuality, 146, 149, 153–154, 194
  transference issues, 148, 151–155
Case of Mr. T, 15–39
  countertransference issues, 26, 229–231
  dreams, 23, 25–26, 28–29, 32–35, 212–214
  factors affecting analyzability, 23–25, 39
  fears of death, 34
  free association, 24, 39
  narcissistic issues, 24, 39
  sexuality, 32–39
  termination, 35–38
  transference issues, 25–31, 35, 37, 39

Case of Mr. W, 107–143
  countertransference issues, 115, 118, 122, 130–131, 136
  dreams, 109, 113, 116–117, 123–126, 128–129, 131–132, 136–138, 142–143
  factors affecting analyzability, 115–119, 143
  free association, 116
  impact of job loss, 107, 113
  impact of prior physical illness, 107–108, 113, 133
  sexuality, 108, 138
  transference issues, 120–121, 124–125, 128–129, 132, 139–143
Castration anxiety secondary to decreased intellectual and cognitive functioning, 188–189
  decreased sensory acuity, 184, 239
  decreased sexual attractiveness, 186
  loss of a child, 199–200
  physical illness, 189–190, 195
Cath, S. H., 7
Committee on Psychoanalytic Practice of the American Psychoanalytic Association, ix
Continuing capacity for pleasure, effect on analyzability, See Analyzability of the older patient
Countertransference feelings toward older patients,
  anger aroused by patients' dependency feelings and/or envy, 4, 7, 226–228
  as a reason for the paucity of clinical data on older patients, x–xii
  as a result of unresolved hostility to one's parents, 4
  as a result of the sexuality of the older patient, 6, 151
  intensity of, 11–12
  Ms. B, 87–93, 99, 102
  Mrs. N, 52, 54–55, 58
  Mrs. R, 148, 151
  Mr. T, 26, 229–231
  Mr. W, 115, 118, 122, 130–131, 136
  Professor F, 161, 163
  resolution by means of the therapist's dreams, 228, 229–235, 243
  therapist's rescue fantasies, 24, 29, 115, 159, 229–231

Daydreams about the past, 8
Death,
  approximations of, 215–216, 242
  as annihilation of the self, 216, 220
  as castration, 3, 216, 219–220
  as claustrophobic equivalent, 216, 218
  as masochistic surrender, 216–217
  as retaliation for destructive impulses, 216–217
  as separation or abandonment, 216, 221
  coming to terms with death, 215–222, 237
  consistent generalizations about death, 215–216, 242
  dreams of death, 5, 171
  fears of death, 4–6, 9–10
  reminiscing as a means of preparing for death, 8
  termination of therapy as an equivalent of death, 5, 217–218
  wish for a younger therapist to remain alive, 27–29, 65, 126, 221–222

Defenses,
    modifications in older patients, 4, 7, 11
    weakening of defenses in narcissistic patients in older age period, 13, 171-172
Dependency needs in older patients, 7, 195-197, 207
Diamond, L., xii
Dreams,
    as a denial of death, 5
    mourning and separation dreams, 49-51, 207-214, 241-242
    of Ms. B, 83-85, 95, 105, 209
    of Mrs. N, 49-51, 57-58, 209-210
    of Mrs. R, 152-153, 210-211, 218-219
    of Mr. T, 23, 25-26, 28-29, 32-35, 212-214
    of Mr. W, 109, 113, 116-117, 123-126, 128-129, 131-132, 136-138, 142-143
    resolution of countertransference problems by means of the therapist's dreams, 228, 229-235, 243. *See also* Countertransference feelings toward older patients
Drives,
    changes in intensity of the drives in older people, 7-8, 193-195, 200-201, 240
Duration of treatment in older patients, 1, 3, 6-8

"Empty nest" syndrome, impact on the older person, 198-203
    how nest was emptied, 198-200
    life-timing of emptying, 198-200, 240
    on feelings of helplessness, passivity, and loss of control, 201-202
    on object-relationships, 240
    on redistribution of drive energy, 200-201, 240. *See also* Drives, changes in intensity of the drives in older people
Envy in older patients, of children and of therapist's youth, 4-5, 9, 12-13, 170-171, 174, 196, 222, 238
Erikson, E. H., 5-6, 170

Feasibility of analytic treatment for patients over the age of 50, ix-x, 237
Fliess, R., 226-227
Fliess, W., 224
Free association, ability of older patients to utilize it, 2-3, 24, 39, 51, 116, 147-149, 155, 160
Freud, S., x, 1, 223-226, 237

Giambra, L. N., 8
Gill, M. M., 225
Gill, M. M., and Hoffman, I. Z., 225
Gitelson, M., 8, 226-227
Goldfarb, A. I., 7
Greenacre, P., 224
Greenson, R. R., 224
Grotjahn, M., 3-4, 6, 170

Heimann, P., 226-227
Hoffer, W., 226-227
Hurn, H. T., 10
Hysterectomy, significance in older patients, 42, 69, 79, 81, 176, 184-185

Identifications,
    complementary, 228
    concordant, 228

Imaginal Process Inventory, 8
Imaginary companion fantasies, 72–73, 82–83
Integrity, concept of, 5–6, 170

Jacques, E., 9, 171

Kaufman, I., 6–7
Kaufman, M. P., 2–3
Kernberg, O. F., 4, 7, 12–13, 171–172, 180, 227, 233
King, P., 11–12, 172, 180, 238
Klein, M., 6, 9, 170
Kohut, H., 10, 225

Langs, R. J., 227, 229
Last chance idea, motivational boost for therapy from patient's awareness of growing older, 11, 23–24, 66–67, 172, 180, 238
Levin, S., 6–7, 170
Linden, M. E., 7
Little, M., 226–227
Losses of aspects of the self
    developmental issues, xi
    impact of losses on the sense of the self, 181–190
    loss of athletic skills, 181–183
    loss of sensory acuity, 183–184
    loss of reproductive or sexual capacity, 184–186
    loss of sexual attractiveness, 186–188
    loss of intellectual and cognitive functioning, 188–189
    physical illness, 189–190
    need to mourn aspects, 5–6, 9, 11, 13

Masturbation in the older person, 22, 32, 61, 63, 65, 96, 155, 186–189, 194, 201

McMahon, A. W., and Rhudick, P. J., 8
Meerloo, J. A. M., 4–5, 170
Memories, recovery of childhood ones in older patients, 5, 10, 237
Myers, W. A., 83, 153, 222, 224

Narcissistic issues in older people
    idealization of the analyst, 10
    losses of the narcissistic investment in the self, 3, 4, 7
    narcissistic investment in athletic skills, 178–179, 181
    narcissistic investment in sexual attractiveness, 186–187
    narcissistic investment in sexual and reproductive capacity, 185
    need for narcissistic personalities to accept limitations of the self, 238
    normal and pathological narcissism, 12–13
    problems narcissistic personalities have in dealing with aging and death, 4
    use of devaluation of others as a defense against envy, 13
    weakening of narcissistic defenses, 13, 170–172
Neugarten, B. L., 9–10, 171
NIMH Conference on Aging, ix

Object loss, 6–8, 12, 170, 172, 175, 183–185, 205–214, 237
    factors in dealing with, 205–214
    loss of athletic skills acquired in relationship to important objects and intensification in fantasy of sense of object loss, 183

Object loss (*continued*)
  loss of reproductive capacity and fear of, 185
  loss of sensory acuity and fear of, 184

Physical illness in older people, 8, 157, 177, 189–190, 195
Population groups underserved by psychoanalysis, adults over 50, ix
Potency problems in older patients, 15–39, 157–167, 172–173, 185–186, 239
Primal scene, 96–97, 146, 151
Prior psychotherapeutic intervention, effect on analyzability, 15–16, 23, 147–149, 172, 178

Racker, H., 227–228
Regression to earlier libidinal positions in the older person, 7
Reich, A., 226–227
Retirement, impact of, xi, 7–8, 191–203
  how work stoppage occurred, 191–193
  life-timing, 191–193
  on feelings of helplessness and passivity, 192–194, 197–198, 240
  on object-relationships, 196–198, 240
  on redistribution of drive energy, 193–195, 240
  on self-esteem, 192–195, 198, 240
Reminiscing in older people, 8
Ross, D. W., and Kapp, F. T., 228

Sandler, A. M., 10–11, 172, 238
Searles, H., 227
Segal, H., 5, 9

Self-esteem, factors affecting it in the older individual
  empty nest syndrome, 198–203
  feelings of loss of control of one's life, 192–194, 197–198, 206
  increased dependency needs, 195–197
  loss of a child, 199, 202
  loss of athletic skills, 181–183, 239
  loss of intellectual and cognitive functioning, 188–189, 239
  loss of object-relationships, 196–198, 206
  loss of reproductive or sexual capacity, 184–186, 239
  loss of sensory acuity, 183–184, 239
  loss of sexual attractiveness, 186–188, 239
  masturbation, 187–189
  physical illness, 189–190, 195, 239
  retirement, 6, 8, 206
Sexuality in the older individual
  countertransference problems of younger therapists, 6
  examples, 8, 22, 32–39, 59–61, 63–65, 78–79, 95–98, 101–102, 106, 108, 138, 146, 149, 153–155, 158, 161–162, 186–189, 194
  redistribution of drive energy, 185, 187, 193–195, 200–201. *See also* Drives, changes in intensity of the drives in older people, 193–195, 200–201, 240
Shainess, N., 11
Strachey, J., 27

Termination of therapy in the older patient
  difficulties in doing, 211–212
  equivalence with death, 217–218

Time, changed perception of it in the older person, 9
Tower, L. E., 228
Transference issues in older patients
  as resistance to recovery of childhood memories, 224–225
  erotic and erotized, 194, 224–225, 238
  intensity of transference, 3–4, 11
  Ms. B, 83, 85–93, 98, 103–104
  Mrs. N, 50–51, 53–56, 58–61, 64, 67
  Mrs. R, 148, 151–155, 194, 225, 238
  Mr. T, 25–31, 35, 37, 39
  Mr. W, 120–121, 124–125, 128–129, 132, 139–143, 225
  narcissistic aspects, 9
  negative transference, 224
  parental and filial transferences, 5
  Professor F, 162
  reluctance of some therapists to interpret transference, 11
  reversed oedipal transference, 4, 6
  similarity to adolescence, 11
Transference neurosis in older patients, 193, 223–224
Treatability of the older patient, evaluation of, 169–180

Winnicott, D. S., 226–227
Wolff, K., 10
Working alliance, 224

Zinberg, N. E., and Kaufman, I., 6